"The Life Coach's Tool Kit, Vol. 2 *isn't just another dry textbook. Imagine it: wisdom distilled from the trenches of real-life coaching, shared by passionate experts from all corners of the globe. Whether you're a seasoned coach seeking fresh inspiration or a newbie eager to ignite your practice, this book is your treasure map to transformation. The Life Coach's Tool Kit, Vol. 2 is waiting to be your partner in this incredible journey.*"

—CLAUDIA SCHEFFLER-PERRONE,
Owner of KillerPress.com, Executive Coach

"*Packed with insights and activities,* The Life Coach's Tool Kit, Vol. 2 *empowers coaches to elevate their practice. Drawing from diverse experts, this essential guide provides techniques to build strong client relationships, facilitate growth, and unlock potential. An invaluable addition to any coach's tool kit.*"

—SVEN GADE, Founder of LeaderTrip Coaching, Inc., Professional Certified Coach

"The Life Coach's Tool Kit, Vol. 2 *holds collective wisdom and practical tools from an impressively diverse group of coaches focusing on various aspects of life. Whether you are a seasoned coach or a brand new one, this condensed overview of a wide range of exercises is an invaluable resource to enhance and enrich your own offering. Whether you're looking for a coach or would like to get a sense of what it's like to work with one, this book will be a solid start.*"

—ELENA KIM, Expert on Community, Workshop Facilitator

"The Life Coach 2 *is chock full of useful coaching tools and unique-coach approach stories from seasoned professionals from all over the world. If you are looking for an understanding of what coaching is all about, this is a great resource with wonderful ways to be able to coach yourself and to use when coaching others. As a professional coach who loves tools, I highly recommend this book as a great resource. It will give you many new approaches to try with your coaching clients and inspire you to share your own story to help others on their way!*"

—GAVAN AMBROSINI, MA PCC, Executive and Leadership Coach, ICF Mentor Coach, Accredited Coaching Supervisor

"The Life Coach's Tool Kit *is a great guide for coaches to easily add a variety of activities into their coaching practice. The wide range of perspectives from multiple co-authors of this book make it a valuable resource for life coaches.*"

—SHAWN FECHTER, Best-selling Co-author of *Peak Performance: Mindset Tools for Sales*

"*There are few better feelings than helping make someone's life better. Life coaches know this firsthand.* The Life Coach's Tool Kit, Vol. 2 *is a terrific source for Life Coaches. Twenty-five international expert coaches share their insights in this must-read resource. Whether you are a new or seasoned life coach, you'll find something here to make your impact resound for generations.*"

—PAUL DANIELS, JR, Speaker, Advisor, Author, Founder of Peripheral Thinkers™

THE LIFE COACH'S TOOL KIT Vol. 2

Ready-to-Use Strategies, Principles, and Activities

THE LIFE COACH'S TOOL KIT Vol. 2

Authored by:
Erik Seversen, Raman Bhangoo, Katerina Bourdoukou,
Noa Brume, Laurie Cozart, Sylvie Drapeau, Hope Firsel,
Curry Glassell, Magdalena Haver, Alissa Janey, Miranda Jol,
Zelda Okia, MD, Rebecca Olson, Anna Pagliuca, David Pasikov,
Anna Prinz, Mark Reinisch, Marisol Rodriguez, Alisa A. Sanè,
Ya'ara Segal, Judy E. Slater, Holly Smevog, Ryan Spence,
Jake Stahl, Julie Stévigny, Diana Usher

THIN LEAF PRESS | LOS ANGELES

The Life Coach's Took Kit, Vol. 2 Copyright © 2024 by Erik Seversen.
All rights reserved. No part of this publication may be reproduced, distributed, or transmitted in any form or by any means, including photocopying, recording, or other electronic or mechanical methods, without the prior written permission of the author, except in the case of brief quotations embodied in reviews and certain other non-commercial uses permitted by copyright law. The contributing authors maintain all rights to use the material inside the chapter he or she wrote for this book.

The Life Coach's Took Kit, Vol. 2 individual chapters. Copyright © 2024 by Raman Bhangoo, Katerina Bourdoukou, Noa Brume, Laurie Cozart, Sylvie Drapeau, Hope Firsel, Curry Glassell, Magdalena Haver, Alissa Janey, Miranda Jol, Zelda Okia, Rebecca Olson, Anna Pagliuca, David Pasikov, Anna Prinz, Mark Reinisch, Marisol Rodriguez, Alisa A. Sanè, Ya'ara Segal, Judy E. Slater, Holly Smevog, Ryan Spence, Jake Stahl, Julie Stévigny, Diana Usher

Disclaimer—The advice, guidelines, and all suggested material in this book is given in the spirit of information with no claims to any particular guaranteed outcomes. This book does not replace professional consultation. Anyone deciding to add physical or mental exercises to their life should reach out to a licensed medical doctor, therapist or consultant before following any of the advice in this book. The authors, publisher, editor, and organizers do not assume and hereby disclaim any liability to any party for any loss, damage, or disruption caused by anything written in this book.

Library of Congress Cataloging-in-Publication Data
Names: Seversen, Erik, Author, et al.
Title: *The Life Coach's Tool Kit, Vol. 2*
LCCN: 2024901706

ISBN 978-1-953183-47-7 (hardcover) | 978-1-953183-46-0 (paperback)
ISBN 978-1-953183-45-3 (eBook) | 978-1-953183-48-4 (audiobook)
Non-Fiction, Coaching, Self-Help, Personal-Development
Cover Design: 100 Covers
Interior Design: Formatted Books
Editor: Nancy Pile
Thin Leaf Press
Los Angeles

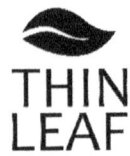

Thank you for reading this book. There are tools found within the following pages that can greatly benefit your life, but don't stop there. Make sure you get the most you can from this book and reach out directly to the expert-authors who want to help you reach your goals by becoming the best life coach you can be and to manifest success in your life. Contact information for each author is found at the end of their respective chapter.

To the pioneer life coaches who have positively transformed lives and to those pursuing to do the same.

CONTENTS

INTRODUCTION XVII
By Erik Seversen
Author of *Ordinary to Extraordinary* and *Explore*
Los Angeles, California

CHAPTER 1
UNLOCKING THE CONVERSATION: BUILDING TRUST AND OPENING DOORS 1
By Raman Bhangoo
Academic Life Coach, ICF Member
Vancouver, British Columbia, Canada

CHAPTER 2
LIFE COACHING THROUGH MINDFULNESS, CREATIVITY, AND COMMUNICATION 9
By Katerina Bourdoukou, MA, MSc
Life & Professional Development Coach
Athens, Greece

CHAPTER 3
INTEGRATING LIFE COACHING TECHNIQUES FOR HOLISTIC PERSONAL DEVELOPMENT 19
By Noa Brume, MBACP
Founder, The International Coaching & Counselling Institute
The Hague, Netherlands

CHAPTER 4
THE TRANSFORMATIVE POWER OF SHIFTING PERSPECTIVES 29
By Laurie Cozart, MBA, MCC, MCNLP
CEO and Executive Coach, Positive Psychology
Danville, California

CHAPTER 5
THE HEART OF COACHING: ACTIVE LISTENING AND ASSESSMENTS 43
By Sylvie Drapeau
Intuitive Life Coach in Personal Development, Author
Montreal, Quebec, Canada

CHAPTER 6
COACHING TOOL KIT 55
By Hope Firsel
Life and Fertility Coach, Rapid Resolution Therapy
Highland Park, Illinois

CHAPTER 7
THE POWER OF ASKING A QUESTION 63
By Curry Glassell
Mentor and Life Coach
Houston, Texas

CHAPTER 8
THE POWER OF KNOWING—SPIRITUAL COACHING WITH PSYCHEDELICS 75
By Magdalena Haver
Spiritual Life Coach, Psychedelic Guide & Facilitator
Amsterdam, The Netherlands

CHAPTER 9
ACHIEVING GOALS WITH THE POWER OF THE FIVE WHYS 87
By Alissa Janey
Author, Life Coach, Creator of ElevateRadiate.com
Minneapolis, Minnesota

CHAPTER 10
MEET ME IN THE MIDDLE: INNER ALIGNMENT AS FREE MEDICINE 99
By Miranda Jol (BSc: Joy of Life)
Owner, Magnetic Vibes; Life Coach
Amersfoort, Netherlands

CHAPTER 11
THE TRANSFORMATIONAL GUIDE TO FLOURISHING PERSONALLY AND PROFESSIONALLY 109
By Zelda Okia, MD
Life and Weight Loss Coach, Forensic Pathologist
Milwaukee, Wisconsin

CHAPTER 12
AN INSIDE-OUT APPROACH TO WORK-LIFE BALANCE 119
By Rebecca Olson
Life Coach for Working Moms, Podcast Host
Benicia, California

CHAPTER 13
NAVIGATING EARLY ADULT LIFE TRANSITIONS 129
By Anna Pagliuca, MSc
Life and Mental Health Coach
Utrecht, Netherlands

CHAPTER 14
TRANSFORMING STRESS INTO STRENGTH: INSIGHTS AND STRATEGIES FOR COACHES 137
By David Pasikov
Executive, Business, and Life Coach, Psychotherapist
Big Rapids, Michigan

CHAPTER 15
CULTIVATING TRANSFORMATIONAL COACHING: HARNESSING THE POWER OF VISION AND VALUES 147
By Anna Prinz
Life Coach; Founder of *The Crossroads Coach*
High Wycombe, England, United Kingdom

CHAPTER 16
VISION-CENTERED COACHING: GUIDING CLIENTS TO DISCOVER THEIR "WHY" ...157
By Mark Reinisch
Author of *The Wellness Ethic*, Life & Transformation Coach
Charleston, South Carolina

CHAPTER 17
COACHING CREATIVELY: GIVING VOICE TO CONFIDENCE 169
By Marisol Rodriguez
Creative Leadership Coach and Facilitator
Chicago, Illinois

CHAPTER 18
MARRIAGE COACHING 179
By Alisa A. Sanè
CEO & Founder of 90 Day Health and Life Coach, Author
Arlington, Tennessee

CHAPTER 19
LEADING WITH LOVE..187
By Ya'ara Segal, CPCC
Life Coach & Trainer for Social Impact
Zurich, Switzerland

CHAPTER 20
UNITING SPIRITUALITY, HEALTH, AND CREATIVE EXPRESSION FOR PERSONAL GROWTH 199
By Judy E. Slater
CEO of Innerlude & Associates, Life Coach
Novato, California

CHAPTER 21
THE CAREER FULFILLMENT ACCELERATOR—FOR COACHING CLIENTS NAVIGATING A CAREER CHANGE 209
By Holly Smevog, MS, ACC
Founder, HMS Consulting, Career & Life Coach
Portland, Maine

CHAPTER 22
CURIOSITY DIDN'T KILL THE CAT, AND IT WON'T KILL YOU 223
By Ryan Spence
Integrative Life Coach, Author of *The Triple C Method*®
Sheffield, England, United Kingdom

CHAPTER 23
THE 2/10 RULE OF EFFECTIVE COMMUNICATION 233
By Jake Stahl
Founder & CEO of Jake Stahl Consulting
Norwich, Connecticut

CHAPTER 24
THE POWER TO TAP INTO YOUR AUTHENTIC SELF 247
By Julie Stévigny
Holistic Life Coach, Author of *Love You Latte, Sophie*
Lievegem, Belgium

CHAPTER 25
THE EM DASH 255
By Diana Usher
All About We, LLC
Lifestyle Management Coach
Oklahoma, USA

DID YOU ENJOY THIS BOOK? 267

INTRODUCTION

By Erik Seversen
Author of *Ordinary to Extraordinary* and *Explore*
Los Angeles, California

The alarm clock sounds loudly, and I struggled to find it in the dark as I was jolted awake from a deep sleep having gone to bed a bit later than I had planned. After a quick shower, I downed a bowl of Frosted Flakes cereal before heading out the door. A quick stop at Starbucks on the way to work provided a mocha-latte which motivated me to start my day. I knew my son had a school volleyball game at 3PM. It was on my calendar since the start of the season, but as the day progressed, and I scarfed down a burger and fries from the local fast-food joint, I became aware that I'd have to miss this one because of a work-related deadline. After a late dinner with my wife, I wanted to do my workout, but felt exhausted. I decided to watch some TV with a beer to relax and ended up staying up a bit too late once again.

The alarm clock sounds loudly, and I struggled to find it in the dark… Here we go again…

The above situation isn't a direct example of my daily life a number of years ago, but it isn't far off either. And, I think it is a very good example of how millions of people live their lives every single day. There is a better way, but without a person deciding to get out from their monotonous (and unhealthy) routine, creating a change in life can be difficult. But it doesn't have to be. Enter the life coach.

With a good life coach, the daily routine doesn't have to be a trudge through life. How does this sound: I woke up two minutes before my opportunity clock would sound, and I reached over and turned it off before it

Introduction

made a noise. I showered thanking God for another day ahead. I meditated for 15 minutes and ate a bowl of oatmeal flavored with blueberries as opposed to the extremely sugary cereal. I also made a simple cup of coffee that didn't cost $5.50 at Starbucks. Since I knew my son had a 3PM volleyball game, I completed a project for my work deadline before lunch, which was a salmon salad. After the volleyball game, I exercised for 45 minutes as was my routine before dinner. After dinner, I sat at the table talking with family for a bit, watched a bit of TV without the beer, read in bed for a few minutes before turning out the lights at 10PM, much earlier than was my previous routine.

So, what is better about this second scenario? Well, everything including better sleep, better nutrition, better time-management, better quality time with family, better financial control, better overall mindset, and ultimately a better way of existing. Really, the changes aren't that drastic, however making a change requires a choice.

In my opinion, making a major change in the way we are living our lives is possible for anyone with or without the help from another person. Having said that, I also think it is very, very difficult to do this alone. Thankfully, we are living in an age whereby attention to how we live our lives is becoming more and more important. And, the people at the cutting edge of this phenomenon are life coaches.

Just like people, there is no one-size-fits-all life coach. Rather, there are those who specialize in weight and nutrition, strength and fitness, business, management, leadership, spiritual awareness, mindful practices, meditation, overcoming trauma and anxiety, marriage and child-raising, transitioning career or other life event, etc. However, with all of these very diverse arenas of life coaching, there is a common thread that the coaching client's life becomes somehow better.

As life coaches, we are helping transform individuals, which helps transform families and workplaces, which helps transform the world, even if a tiny bit. Yes, life coaches are making the world a better place. If you look at many of the changes happening over the past twenty years, you can clearly see a better awareness of people living intentionally and striving to live their best lives. Twenty-five years ago, meditation in the workplace, yoga in the school system, and even a healthy balance between corporate and family life were rare. Now, we're seeing these things as common, but there is still a long way to go. There are still millions of people who are not getting the help they need. This is one of the reasons I'm so excited about producing Vol. 2 of *The Life Coach's Tool Kit*.

If you read the introduction to *The Life Coach's Tool Kit, Vol. 1*, you've seen that the concept for this book was me thinking to myself, *I wish I had a book filled with different chapters with different ideas from different experts about life coaching. I wish I had a book with simple coaching activities that would work for various situations.* Well, that book was created, and the effect was extraordinary. I'm now happy to offer another volume of tools that life coaches can use to work with their clients in many different situations.

Like *The Life Coach's Tool Kit, Vol. 1*, this book is designed for anyone wanting to learn principles, philosophies, ideas, and activities related to life coaching. This book will be a great resource for new life coaches just starting out who want to be the best they can be. This book will also be great for the seasoned life coach who may have been using the same coaching philosophy for years and who wants to inject a few new ideas into their coaching practice, especially with their long-term clients.

I'm excited to share Vol. 2 of *The Life Coach's Tool Kit* with the world, and I'm excited about the expert authors who contributed to it. For this book, I solicited the help of 25 experts from various backgrounds and locations. The number one goal in *The Life Coach's Tool Kit, Vol 2* is to provide more examples and strategies from elite coaches, mentors, psychologists, doctors, therapists, business owners, authors, and lifestyle experts who all have something unique to say about life coaching.

The experts authoring this book are from all over the USA, Canada, the United Kingdom, the Netherlands, Switzerland, Belgium, and Greece. They are professionals who are leadership, emotional intelligence, and communication experts, senior business executives, hypnotists, wealth and growth coaches, psychedelic experience experts, podcast and radio hosts, TEDx speakers, motivational keynote speakers, military veterans, medical doctors, psychotherapists, marriage experts, C-suite strategists, neuro-linguistic programming masters, retreat facilitators, consultants, and more. The one thing the authors of this book have in common is that they all have an idea about life coaching, and these ideas can be applied to multiple life coaching situations. These ideas are available to you now.

Although this book is organized around the united theme of mindset and peak performance for life coaches, each chapter is totally stand-alone.

Introduction

The chapters in the book can be read in any order. I encourage you to look through the Table of Contents and begin wherever you want. However, I urge you to read all the chapters because, as a whole, they provide a great array of perspectives. The chapters are arranged with a general principle, philosophy, or technique followed by a short activity that coaches should be able to easily review and use with clients. Each chapter is valuable in helping you tap into your full potential by adding unique tools to your life coaching practice and your life.

It is my hope that you discover something in this book that helps take your life coaching performance to the next level, so you can enthusiastically reach new heights as a life coach and rapidly reach your goals—and at the same time assist your clients to do the same.

About the Author

Erik Seversen is on a mission to inspire people. He holds a master's degree in anthropology and is a certified practitioner of neuro-linguistic programming. Erik draws from his years of teaching at the university level and years of real-life experience to motivate people to take action, creating extreme success in business and in life.

Erik is a TEDx and keynote speaker who has reached over one million people through his public speaking and live courses. He has visited 95 countries and all 50 states in the USA and has climbed the highest mountains on 4 continents, 15 countries, and 18 states. Erik has published thirteen bestselling books on topics of mindset, success, and peak performance, and he has helped over 300 people become best-selling authors. He is a full-time writer, book consultant, and speaker, and he lives by the idea that success is available to everyone—that living an extraordinary life is a choice.

Erik lives in Los Angeles with his wife and two teenage boys.

Contact Erik for interviews, speaking, or book publishing consultation.

Email: Erik@ErikSeversen.com
Website: www.ErikSeversen.com
LinkedIn: https://www.linkedin.com/in/erikseversen/

CHAPTER

1

Unlocking the Conversation: Building Trust and Opening Doors

By Raman Bhangoo
Academic Life Coach, ICF Member
Vancouver, British Columbia, Canada

The most important thing in communication is to hear what isn't being said.

—Peter Drucker

Do you want to know how I get complete strangers to tell me everything about their lives? As I write this, I can see how I sound like a con artist. Let's take the "con" part out; I call this "art." The ability to connect with someone in just a few minutes after meeting them at a level where they feel complete comfort in telling me their deepest fears, passions, and their past history has been a key factor in the success of my coaching.

Now this was not always the case. When I first started coaching, I would be banging my head against a wall. (Imagine the emoji with the brick wall; that was me.) Trying to get my clients to open up was one of my major roadblocks as a new coach. A majority of my clients ranged from high school to college students and also included graduates with newly minted degrees. They were nervous, apprehensive, and didn't trust most people to give them the right advice about which direction to take. As my coaching practice expanded to include adults in all walks of professional life, this common re'action was just as prevalent. The question loomed—Why did I have so much nervous energy around engaging with someone to guide them through the next phase of their journey?

I often enjoy networking events and similar opportunities. The chance to strike up a conversation with new and interesting people can be fun and engaging. For some people, however, this first conversation can feel scary and intimidating, let alone imagining that a deep and genuine connection is even possible. I want to share some practices and a "to-do" list that have really worked for me in breaking that ice as well as what I continue to use in my coaching practice.

Make your client feel like they are the most important person in your world for that one hour you have together. Start with their name, clarify pronunciation and the meaning of their name. How did their parents choose that name? Write down details as they come up: birthdays and any upcoming significant events in their life. I love sending a note to my clients on their birthdays. It's not a sales or promotional tactic, but I know how special it can make someone feel. My kids, to this day, get excited when they get a birthday card in the mail from their dentist.

Genuine interest and curiosity create room for connections, and adding authenticity takes these connections to a deeper level. Recently, I received a random phone call while I was out doing some retail therapy. It was a college student on the line who wanted to talk about body dysmorphia and sounded very nervous. I knew it must have taken a lot of courage for this young man to make the connection. I let him know I was not in a place where I could talk, but I set up a time for later that day. When we connected, I listened while being mindful that I did not have a great deal of experience with this topic. I gave him the space to educate me on his background, and he disclosed the mental distress this situation had caused him. I asked him further questions to understand the exact problem. Long story short, this was a situation that needed to be addressed by a mental health counselor, so I coached him on how to connect with the right people.

A few weeks later, I received a message from this student expressing his gratitude for the time I took to understand him and learn more about him. That one phone call, he said, had made a drastic and positive change in his life. Asking open-ended questions and asking for clarification when there was uncertainty on my end were what this individual needed to help shape his own process of reflection and understanding. I asked for clarification on things I did not know, and I asked for specific examples that led to discovering what this individual needed.

The right word may be effective, but no word was ever as effective as a rightly timed pause.
—Mark Twain

The power of silence cannot be underestimated. The inclination has always been to fill spaces of silence with words, but what I have noticed is that often, a creative shift can happen when someone is given time for thought and reflection. The result can be fascinating and at times can take the client by surprise as we continue to move the conversation forward.

The practice of being vulnerable with my clients helps create a more humanistic connection. One of the biggest misunderstandings that new coaches have is that they should know everything and provide advice. In fact, coaching is a collaborative process where you can show or share examples of vulnerability in the service of a client's growth and well-being. As much as you may feel pressure as a coach to deliver a "perfect" session with your client, the most important thing is to create a safe and empathetic space for them to explore their own vulnerabilities and challenges.

One time, I was engaged in helping a client address the overuse of social media. It was clear she wanted to overcome this situation that prevented her from doing anything productive. She came down hard on herself and felt she was disappointing her parents. I shared my own story with her on how my kids told me that sometimes I am on my phone too much and only "half listening" to them. Immediately, I could see the relief in her face as she told me she didn't realize this was also a problem amongst adults. She went on to ask me how old my kids were, and we discovered that she and my daughter were involved in the same type of dance. These extra few minutes of sharing my personal story deepened our connection, and my client felt even more comfortable opening up afterwards.

Now that we have tackled some practices used to build relationships, how do we take it to the next level? This is where listening comes in. Earlier I mentioned that I have an easy time connecting with people and don't fear initial conversations, but I really had to learn deep listening skills. Indeed, each one of us has the ability to become a better listener. It was something that my husband said that made me realize I am a talker but not the best listener. We had a group of friends over for dinner and the conversation was flowing really well, and the next morning, I said to my husband that it was such a great night. Now my husband is more of the observer, and he said, "You know, sometimes you need to take a breath when talking." I asked him what he meant, and he said that there were many missed opportunities where had I listened, I could've learned more about what was going on in my friends' lives. I was stunned. I thought my being social and chatty was always seen as a positive, so I started observing my own self and had an aha moment: I need to learn to become a better and deeper listener. Here are some practices that have helped enhance my listening skills.

When someone is speaking, have you ever noticed that you are thinking about what you are going to say next? By doing this, you may be missing some key moments in the conversation. If you listen to understand instead of plotting your next response, you can gather important information to formulate powerful and direct questions, guiding and coaching your client to a solution. If you start to lose focus, come back, make eye contact, and lean into your clients' words. This takes practice, but over time, you will notice that you are more present and engaged in what the other person is saying.

There was a client I had been coaching for a while who mentioned the date of a big test that he was preparing for. He expressed how anxious he was feeling. As we talked, I scribbled down the date as I knew we did not have any more sessions lined up since he wanted to focus on his studying. A few days before his test, I reached out and wished him well on his upcoming test and reminded him of the tools we had worked on to help him overcome anxiety. He was so happy that I remembered, and he called me after his exam to say that the message had really "pumped him up." He was able to go into the test with a focused mindset and use some of the methods we had discussed to overcome anxiety. Often, it is small details that I take note of with clients that can become important ways of helping them bolster behaviors while navigating forward with confidence.

Have you noticed when you ask someone, "How are you doing?" that most of the time you get, "I'm good, how are you?" But, if you ask, "No, but how are you REALLY doing?" you will generally get a better response when your client opens up. I was meeting a client one afternoon whom I had not seen for a few weeks. I asked her how things were going, and she replied "good." When I asked again and emphasized "really," she got emotional and let everything spill on the depression she'd been experiencing: the strain on her marriage and the challenges she'd been dealing with overall. It had only been a few weeks since I had seen her but so much had changed, and I was not expecting all that she shared. On numerous occasions, asking this question again with an emphasis on "really" has pivoted the conversation in a meaningful direction.

Letting go of a rigid format of questions and having an open dialogue often ensure we can get more out of a conversation. The other "hat" I often wear is that of an HR professional in the area of recruitment. Some of the best interviews I have conducted often included a conversational flow as opposed to a linear question-and-answer format. In a conversational setting I have found candidates are relaxed and are able to give more in-depth answers with examples instead of what the interviewer may want to hear. I have applied this same approach in my coaching practice and it works really well. You can do this too.

ACTIVITY

The High School Student Wheel of Life

Relationship building and listening skills are only the starting points. A great exercise while doing a discovery or initial consultation with your clients is called the Wheel of Life. I learned this during my coaching program and continue to use this activity to date. The Wheel of Life is a great visual that gives a coach a quick snapshot of their client's life and what areas need to be focused on during coaching.

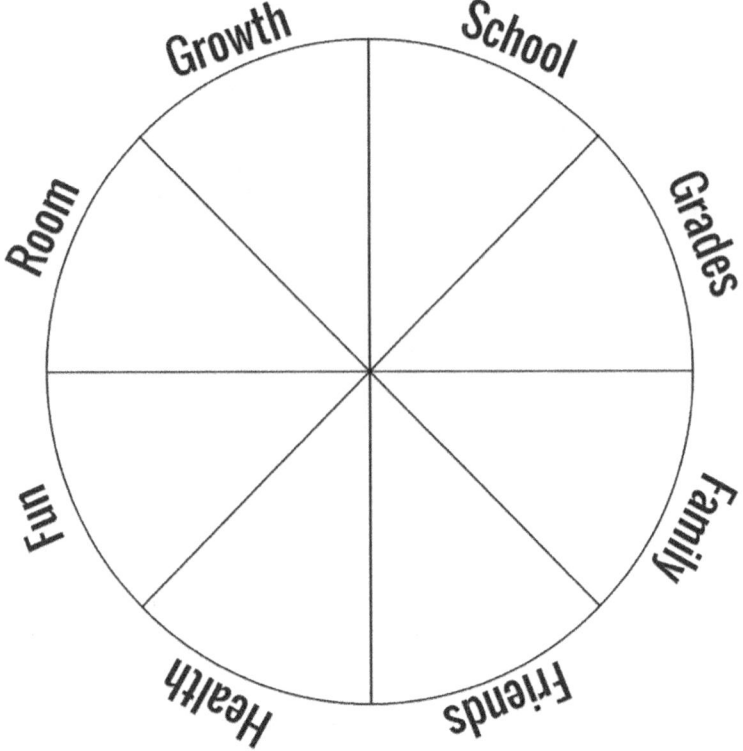

Here are important categories when coaching high school students. Ask a client to draw a circle with these categories and have them rate each category from one to ten on their current level of satisfaction in each area. From this exercise, coaches can generate insights into a client's current life and what matters most. Some questions to get the conversation going with a client can be the following:

1. What jumps out at you when you look at your wheel?
2. If you were to choose just one wedge to tell me more about, which one would you like to discuss?
3. In your chosen wedge, what is one action that would increase the number from 6 to 7 (for instance)?
4. What do you feel are some action steps you can take to move forward?

You can, of course, change the categories based on your client. It is recommended to do this activity in your initial coaching sessions and then again in the very last session. It's a very powerful tool for the client to see how they have progressed in their coaching journey.

As you continue to master your relationship building and listening skills, you will be in a position to quickly uncover what matters most in your client's situation, so you can effectively guide and add value as a coach. It is important to work on improving these skills; oftentimes, the best people to practice with are your family and friends. When listening tools are used effectively, it can take your coaching practice to the next level.

About the Author

Raman Bhangoo is an accomplished and certified life coach through the International Coaches Federation. Her purpose is to connect with youth, teens, and university/college students to help them overcome any personal or academic hurdles to empower them to see their full potential, draw on their passions, and lead a life filled with success and happiness. She often gets invited to do workshops in schools, and she provides her expertise on radio and interviews professionals on her careers podcast.

In addition to coaching students worldwide, she is an HR professional and provides career coaching to a wide range of individuals who are at various stages of their career journey.

When she's not coaching, Raman can be found walking or biking the seawall or hiking the many trails of her hometown in Vancouver, British Columbia.

Email: raman@path2successcoaching.com
Website: www.path2successcoaching.com

CHAPTER 2

Life Coaching through Mindfulness, Creativity, and Communication

By Katerina Bourdoukou, MA, MSc
Life & Professional Development Coach
Athens, Greece

Concerning all acts of initiative and creation, there is one elementary truth, the ignorance of which kills countless ideas and splendid plans: that the moment one definitely commits oneself, then Providence moves too.

—W. H. Murray

Let us consider this hypothesis: You move back to a time several years ago; a person is in a small apartment; the days appear all similar, coming and going with these repetitive gray shades; the room walls appear heavy and monotonous, causing states of anger, despair, and dissatisfaction. Move on some years later; this person is in a room, enjoying a cup of morning coffee; a layer of sun enters the window. This human being is journaling infinite tiny moments of gratitude, pursues music lessons, and studies to improve business skills and human relationships.

You were able read the above story in a few seconds though for the person in the story, it required many small steps to light an unknown area of life. There were lots of hills to walk till she reached a high mountain of light. Numerous preparation sessions happened before making a series of decisions and actions to bring out a change. She had to make many attempts at crossing a little lake before crossing an ocean and feeling the light.

For changes like the above to happen, there are some core ingredients, which lead to the holistic change. These include a total perception of body, mind, soul, and spirit unity and a harmonious state of being. It starts with some powerful vocabulary patterns that stimulate the alteration that leads to magnificent states of gratitude and peaceful-mind responsiveness. While working with clients, I share concepts after working long-term on gratitude in theory and practice. This progressively unleashes imagination and creativity and cultivates a fertile ground of newborn, reconsidered communication.

In this chapter, I unfold a story of fulfillment created from tiny bits of purposeful satisfaction moments to inspiring waves of blessed and empathetic interactions, analogous to the modern interpretation of the butterfly effect. The growth mindset I highlight can be penetrated by an intention with humility that sends out a whole new manifestation, giving the baton to an empathetic sense of empowerment passed from human to human. There are four areas I'd like to cover.

1. Immersing in a Mindful Universe: A Mindful Approach and the Power of Positive Words

Think—Feel—Be

These three words synthesized my motto in the year 2019. It was one morning during a period in which I was attending lots of trainings and webinars. At the same time, I was performing a series of practical exercises to bring out remarkable changes. I remember that day, I woke up, slightly opened my eyes, saw a little light entering from the window, and then it came, as if my world of ideas whispered it to me. "Think—Feel—Be." Years of study, research, work, and exercising was summarized in three words.

The power of these simple words showed how I could communicate the message that a single thought has the potential to produce meaning and that this meaning has a strong impact. The thought one individual chooses to pursue produces a relevant result. Back in 2013, I was unhappy, but taking a friend's positive life transformation into account, I said to myself, "The world around me will not change if I do not change myself." So I started doing things to convince myself that I could achieve the results I wanted. In changing strategies, I could expect diverse outcomes. I made the decision to work in the Greek hotel industry. Simultaneously, I subscribed as a member and worked part-time in a multinational business organization, where I had to set up programs to help people control their weight. I was also in charge of the sales of relevant products to facilitate the procedure to achieve their goals. Within this framework, I attended numerous training sessions and collaborated with various people. It was at this point that I was advised to read a couple of books and start performing relevant exercises to adopt healthy habits and improve my well-being.

I was practicing gratitude exercises every day. Every day, I wrote a list of ten simple elements, which made me grateful. Those were objects like my bed, my cover, or my window. Other things like my small apartment, my people, my coffee, and homemade food came next. Later, I started including elements such as degrees I had obtained or successful moments at work. I suggest that you attempt applying such exercises in your everyday life and encourage your clients to do the same. You may find your own causes to be grateful for, such as things, moments, or people. You may even create a list of ten happy moments from your childhood, family life, social life, or business life. You may take some minutes to review your lists every day so that you can increase the gratitude magnitude of your life. You may also empower your clients to act similarly, discovering their own unique gratitude journey. In my experience I have seen first-hand the power of gratitude. The exercise I give you at the end of the chapter is essentially connected with this panorama of gratitude.

After several years of physical application, I began to be able to connect faster with my body, my feelings, and my inner world. Thoughts and emotions were instantly cooperating to be one. I had created a friendly connection with my body, with my actual self. At this point came the next phase: "Connect—Embody—Transform." That would represent connection, embodiment of desired positive states and a vital, holistic transformation. Later, I became aware of the message of "Feel—Flow—Free," representing a path of emotion trainings, which would lead to a flow in various aspects of life with a sense of internal freedom, characterized by a deeper perception of maintaining the measure concerning the planning and realization of higher achievements.

I would encourage you to reflect on these three-word-clusters. Furthermore, I would suggest you work deeply with yourself and find three verbs, which stimulate the journey of your transformation. You may also work on this scenario with your clients using any of the three-verb series. Discovering your own or your clients' three power verbs can shape a personal path of transformation and fulfillment.

Certification in life coaching was an unveiling procedure. I had already collected lots of exercises, practices, and outcomes in my notebooks, when in 2020, the COVID-19 pandemic came. I made the decision to help more people during this time of a demanding social environment. While working on my life coaching certification, I was also working at a quality- and cost-control department in a catering business. However, I was immersed in this coaching journey. Applying simple exercises had progressively brought a remarkable change in my life. I deepened the research referring to human nature with coaching tools. With several simple exercises, life coaching can help you perform work tasks more productively while embarking on a unique journey of self-awareness in multiple levels and improving your relationship with yourself and with other people. This element can produce real positive magic and bright miracles.

Speaking about the power of words and mindful consideration, personal branding is a significant attribute you need to handle with particular care. You may use the five-minute exercise described at the end of the chapter to enhance creativity and inspiration before starting to work on the textures, colors, meaning, and vocabulary of your brand. You may dare to propose this alone or with your collaborating teams, or your clients to expand creativity while working with brand features such as purpose, storytelling, and vision.

When you feel prepared enough to continue, then set the plan. Here is a proposed combination of steps SET: "Stimulate—Empower—Thrive." Find and define what is significant for you; do the steps and relevant procedures to adequately empower yourself and others; and let the plan thrive. For example, the eight stimulating ingredients that I connect with my personal branding and professional life are these: emotion awareness and management, training-coaching, arts and culture, decision making, patience, public speaking, volunteering, and feminine energy vibes. These elements have been functioning as fuel, filling me with value and inspiration to continue the journey, serving society through a company and as a volunteer. So, pick up your stimuli, empower yourself and your people, get empowered, and let yourself and your plans thrive.

2. Enhancing Creativity

As my background is in writing and performing arts, I am particularly sensitive with amateur and professional artists. I have seen miracles with the exercise I'll be sharing. I encourage you to customize it to your own circumstance and communicate the approach to other people. Humans who are fond of arts and practice them may use the approach given in the exercise before their rehearsals, to begin the rehearsal or to finish and attain a peaceful state of mind. Some minutes of mindfulness can diminish creative limitations, giving space to bright ideas and freeing the power of physical and vocal expression. Artists of all creative art venues may use the exercise to recharge their psychic and spiritual aspirations, boosting their unique creative potential.

Naturally, the exercise can be incorporated in classes from various fields, everyday life activities that need a glimpse of creativity, demanding business meetings, and diverse learning and development environments. The end-of-chapter exercise offers a beautiful path of infinite creation, positive interaction, and imagination freedom.

3. Smoothing Communications

Life coaching has the tools to contribute to people's upskilling during communications procedures. Those skills contribute to improving the quality of communications in personal, social, and business sectors, helping you create better relationships and build effective teams. Active listening, emotional awareness, time management, effective verbal and written communications, soft skills, and leadership skills lead toward productive communication processes.

You may include the exercise shared at the end of the chapter to improve the aforementioned communication dimensions. For example, concerning active listening, the exercise may help you relax at the beginning of your coaching session. You may perform it by yourself and also with your client so that you have better quality communications during the session and create brilliant outcomes. A relaxed mind is associated with diminishing stress and actively participating with a bigger physical and psychic potential.

The same exercise contributes to improving emotional awareness. It helps you to reach a holistic consideration of time management. Some timetables or time deadlines may cause people stress; it will help doing the five-minute exercise before you set your timetables or during the procedures. When things do not go as expected, take some time to relax and then proceed with a new solution or an alternative option. Once you become familiar with the exercise or if you are already advanced in mindfulness practices, you may attempt to work on more positive emotions for a longer time and expand your expressive palette.

4. Handling Dysfunctional Beliefs—Mindfulness—Manifestation

You may use the end-of-chapter exercise to manage dysfunctional beliefs and focus on the positive side. You need to take into account that, as a human being, you have your personal limiting or dysfunctional beliefs; thus, in most cases, you are able to help clients in the fields that you specialize in, and you have fewer limiting or dysfunctional beliefs than them so you help them progress. In case you want some information or need a reminder referring to the ways we find and define limiting beliefs, I suggest this simple strategy. Review the aspects of your life such as the personal, social, or professional dimensions. You may use the exercise to relax and attain a positive state and then examine the issues that need improvement. For example, your emotional state, your relationships, your community contribution, or your business career. In the fields that you acknowledge that you are "stuck," this is where there are dysfunctional and limiting beliefs to resolve. This exercise is a personified approach to smooth the relationship with yourself or with your clients and progressively uncover hidden potential.

Conclusion

My love for coaching skills arose from the significant, massive, positive transformation I noticed in all aspects of life brought out by practicing the skills. Mindfulness, creativity and communication became lighthouses during my journey, and as a result, I heartily desire to transmit the message to others. Years of study and application brought me to this point after being in numerous destinations and experiencing remarkable encounters with wonderful humans in this world. My most genuine intention is to transmit this meaningful substance of life, which is a spirit of gifted change. Feel free to get inspiration from any of those stimuli and enlighten your deepest, personal, and honest truth to be in contact with your higher purpose and manifest your ideas, visions, and dreams.

ACTIVITY

Exercise for Coaches and Coaching Clients

According to a Harvard publication, 10 to 15 minutes a day of mindfulness practice produces beneficial results, and consistent practice unlocks great potential. Inspired by this, I created this pocket-task to improve participants' concentration, creativity, decision making, problem solving, resilience, wellness, emotional well-being, visualization, mental health nurturing, and performance support.

The milestone tool is a five-minute relaxation and mindfulness time with a focus on positivity. The exercise is for a coach and coachee in one-on-one sessions or for group coaching. It can be performed in person or during online sessions. You may attempt to apply it at the introductory time of your sessions or keep it in your kit as a transformational positive habit and routine.

The activity is simple. Find a comfortable space to be. Focus on your breath. Inhale, then exhale peacefully. The pace is slow. You may close your eyes or keep them open. You may sit or lie on the floor. You may keep your hands on your belly and peacefully feel the movement of your belly. Do this for approximately one minute.

Then, start noticing what happens in your body for the following minute. You may feel that the heartbeat pace slows down. You may feel that more oxygen enters your body, and the blood circulates more freely.

Start noticing your body in the space during the third minute. Where are you located: a chair, a couch, a bed, the floor, or on the earth? Find the connection with the points that support you. Continue feeling your inhale-exhale experience.

Next, in the fourth minute, bring one memory connected with a positive state such as gratitude, love, affection, joy, or happiness. It can be from your current life, from the past, from your childhood. It doesn't matter as long as it's a happiness moment.

Bring your attention to your breath again for the fifth minute. Feel the inhale and exhale of the body process. Notice what happens to your body. How do you feel now? What are the differences, visual or non-visual, from your state before? You may notice a transformation in your body, your facial characteristics, or your wellness state.

Feel free to write about this if you apply it to a session to discuss the states with your coachee(s). Encourage people to describe and talk about the experience.

Note: When you become familiar with the exercise, notice also how your voice transforms, both your own voice and that of your coachee, after the implementation of the task.

Limitations

I encourage you to keep a friendly attitude toward dysfunctional beliefs. Many people quit when things do not go as primarily expected. When this occurs, come back again and again to search for potential limiting beliefs and handle them with positivity and care. Feel your breath, perform the exercise, defend self-awareness, expand a giving spirit, and feed the law of attraction with positive affirmations.

About the Author

Katerina Bourdoukou loves expressing meaningful truthful essences of Life. She graduated from the 1st Lyceum (Highschool) of N. Smyrni Athens Greece. She Studied Communication, Media and Culture, Theatre Studies, Acting and Directing, International Hospitality Management and Life Coaching. Since she was a child, she loved writing and languages. During her BA, she lived for six months in Belgium and for one year she studied in University of London and Royal Academy of Dramatic Art. She likes travelling; thus, she has been in many European Countries and the U.S.A. Katerina is currently working as a Coach and serving as a Learning

Facilitator in various actions. She writes for her blog, creates poems and songs; she contributes also as a creative performer. She is a Volunteer focusing on Education Sector and part of Mentors team in the company 100Mentors.

Email: katerinabourdoukou@gmail.com
LinkedIn: https://www.linkedin.com/in/katerina-bourdoukou
Website(s): www.feminines.gr
www.mindfulharmonyhub.com

CHAPTER 3

Integrating Life Coaching Techniques for Holistic Personal Development

By Noa Brume, MBACP
Founder, The International Coaching & Counselling Institute
The Hague, Netherlands

Are we all coaches? No.
Can we all use the tools and skills coaches use?
Definitely yes.
When coaches hear these three things, their ears catch fire:

1. Everyone calls themselves a coach.
2. Everyone can be a coach.
2. I'm coaching my friends all the time.

While the first two sentences can be argued to be somehow true, and this is what this chapter will come to explain, the third is a complete misunderstanding of the coaching profession. Let me explain.

"Everyone calls themselves a coach nowadays." In many places in the world, "coaching" is considered what we call a "free profession." This means that it is not regulated by the government, and, therefore, technically, everyone can call themselves so. Or as I explain it to my students: Everyone can put a sign on their door saying, "Coach."

So who is regulating these professions?

The professional organisations, federations, and councils, specific to coaching.

They operate a membership scheme into which they only accept members who studied enough and practised enough coaching hours under supervision. They also give accreditation to coaching programmes and write and revise the ethical codes of coaching. In some places, a person can only work as a coach if they have such membership, and in other places, it's actually regulated by the local governing bodies.

I'm happy to say that the more this profession is developing, and the more people appreciate the help they get from coaches, the more recognition is expected. Some organisations and companies will only hire people who are accredited members of a professional body.

But this is actually more acute than that: Coaching is a helping profession. We deal with people's lives. Our work can change someone's way of living, working, behaving, and being. I'll be gutted to think that anyone can think that they can just put a sign on their door and say: "I can help you to change your life, but I have no sufficient education on the matter, but, hey, who cares, it's not illegal to do so, so that's what I'll do."

"Everyone can be a coach." Well, potentially yes. Of course. Everyone who loves working with people and considers themselves what I call a "people-person" has the potential to become a coach.

But let me tell you this: to study coaching takes time, effort, and a huge dedication to the idea of helping others. It means learning to shut down your ego completely and learning to be there for someone else 100%.

It means learning how to change the way you converse, to forget about giving your advice and ideas, and to work day in and day out for the growth and well-being of other people. I know many people who decide to do that, and they do a great job, but both you and I know that coaching is not for everyone.

"I'm coaching my friends all the time."

No, you're not.

It could be that you're a great listener, that you are always the person friends and acquaintances come to open their hearts to and even cry on your shoulder, but this is not coaching. This is being an amazing supporter with a big heart—but not a coaching practitioner.

You see, coaching is a structured way of helping people. It's knowing how to take someone from point A to a more desirable point B in their life. It's setting goals and looking at ways to achieve them. It's empowering other people, and it's working in a constructive way, which can take weeks or months.

And while it is true that listening and empathy are at the heart of it all, we need more than that for the work to be done properly and professionally.

Have I put you off the idea completely?

I really hope not.

Because there's such a huge impact you can make as a coach, it's simply unimaginable that those things are actually not taught in every school in every country. Especially given that schooling has moved away from imparting knowledge because it is there at the tip of a mouse click. Schools should be there to teach students self-sufficiency, how to reflect and adjust their work, how to set and achieve their own goals, how to communicate effectively with others and collaborate as teams, and how to be there for others while accepting them as being there for you.

As AI and instant information further establish their presence in our lives, the importance of essential human skills are crucial in order to get by in this developing world.

Take businesses for example. They heavily rely on sales, customer care, communication, problem-solving, outside-the-box thinking, safety (including emotional safety and well-being to prevent burnout) and more. These are all what used to be called "soft skills," but now the term is changing, and we hear the language of "power skills," "people skills," and "interpersonal skills."

Such skills are related to leadership, productivity, communication, teamwork, and well-being, and are vital to every employee's performance. It is, therefore, not a surprise that the need for those has intensified. I know from a few HR experts that these are the skills they are looking to see in applicants' CVs.

The more automation increases, the more we'll need to use and educate people to use human skills and competencies such as critical and imaginative problem-solving, appropriate communication, emotional intelligence, effective collaboration, and the ability to make complex decisions in the ever-changing work environment.

How can learning coaching help with all that?

In order to answer this question, I thought that the best thing is to pose it to my coaching students. After all, they are the ones who are learning it and can feel the change that training as a coach can bring to someone's life.

I asked the same thing in all the groups: from the foundation level students, all the way to the advanced coach practitioner course students. I also asked the students who I train in organisations because I was curious to see if their answers were similar to the people who chose to train as coaches out of their own personal choice.

I wanted to know the following: How did learning coaching help your personal development, and where did it make the biggest difference for you?

Here's a summary of their answers put into three key points.

I'll start with the answer that surprised me the most, but the more I reflected on the "me" I was before I learnt coaching and the "me" I am now, it made a lot of sense.

1. Coaching Is a Protecting Tool

A protecting tool?

They explained that a huge part of coaching is working on your boundaries. You need to know not only what you are able to do as a coach but also what your competencies are at any given moment in your professional development. What is also very important is to know how to set your professional boundaries in front of clients.

This means a few things:

- Knowing when, where, and how much you are available for clients
- Knowing to help your clients but not become their saviour as they should do that for themselves (super important)
- Learning how not to drain yourself
- Knowing *how* to focus on what's really important and what will help the process to progress the most

- Learning how to, on the one hand, be there 100% present in a situation, and on the other hand, to conserve your energy
- Learning to ask for help

Learning to work with what is right for you and being aware of your capacities and what you can or can't offer can turn you from a person who used to help people at all times (to the point that you might be feeling used), to becoming a person who is aware of their abilities, who knows where and in what way the help is most effective. This will allow you to choose who you help and how much.

The amazing thing that usually happens when you set your boundaries: People appreciate you more.

Because you learnt to say no, you're more energetic, you enjoy the things you do more, and you start to see that people appreciate you more. In fact, they even tell you that they want to learn to do that too, and learn it from you.

Recognising your own best qualities protects you from drainage, burnout, and disappointment, and puts you in control of your decisions and your life. Knowing how to regulate your energy is crucial for your vitality and maintenance of a good and energetic life.

DIY

A good way to protect ourselves is to know well what our values are. Our values determine our priorities, and they're the measures we use to tell if our life is turning out the way we wish. When we know what our values are, it's easier to set boundaries.

In order to know yourself well, it's important to be aware of your values and to reflect and to apply them in daily living. Here's a game you can use with friends and family, revealing personal values. Ask them this: "What will people say about you at your retirement party?"

This will give a great indication as to what's important for you. These are your values.

2. Coaching Helps You to Connect with Others

The world we live in is a world in which there's decreasing personal connection. While we are able to link ourselves to the rest of the world via the internet in seconds, talk to anyone on the planet for free and see them on a video call, we are losing the personal aspect of connection. It seems that the more the world is connected by technology, the more we are disconnected as human beings.

We're social animals. We are mammals and, therefore, thrive on touch and connection. This is how we're being fed as babies, and this is what we're striving for as adults too. It is a known thing that people who have a strong circle of family and friends live longer and are healthier. It's enough to watch *Live to 100: Secrets of the Blue Zones*, a Netflix series by the author Dan Buettner to understand how daily personal connection is crucial for our health, well-being, and longevity.

In coaching, we work on that a lot. There can be no coaching if there's no "coaching relationship" established. This is the foundation of the whole process. Nothing will work or progress if no relationship is established and well-maintained throughout the process.

How is such a relationship created?

By learning and establishing coaching skills that become our second nature. Such skills are listening skills (both active listening and the ability to adapt the way you're listening to the person speaking), empathy, talking at eye level, respect, and building trust.

Connecting to others is relevant to all walks of life: with our partners, children, parents, extended family, neighbours, colleagues, service providers, and more.

Knowing to create a good relationship will fill us with joy, love, happiness, and a sense of belonging.

And it will, as Buettner shows, add to us living longer and feeling better.

DIY

The biggest mistake that people make when they think they're listening is that they're constantly occupying themselves thinking about the response they're about to give. Good listening starts with just hearing the person talking and taking in what they've expressed.

A good way to show them that we've listened carefully is paraphrasing. Paraphrasing is giving reflection on what was said to you. It's repeating back to the person talking to you what you've heard in your own words. Paraphrasing isn't repeating but rather saying what we hear in different words. This does two things:

1. If you're able to repeat, it's clear that you've listened carefully to what was said.
2. It gives your partner the opportunity to "hear" themselves but from another angle, and this can lead to deep reflection.

So here are a few examples for paraphrasing: "When we still lived at home, my parents were helping us a lot. Now things are a mess." Possible paraphrasing:

- "Your parents helped you to keep on top of things."
- "You miss your parents' help."
- "You don't feel in control without your parents' help."

Here's another example: "I'm not sure if I'm ready to take the next step in my career. I feel that I'm lacking some skills." Possible paraphrasing:

- "Your feel that you need more skills in order to move on with your career."
- "You're not sure you're ready to advance at work because of skill level."
- "It sounds like you're wondering if your skills are enough to move on professionally."

You will know when you used paraphrasing well when the person you're talking to will agree with you or show other signs of recognition that they're being understood. Start your paraphrasing with:

- "So what you're saying is…"
- "What I hear you sharing is…"
- "Sounds like you…"

3. With Coaching, You Experience Self-awareness and Self-love

Coaches are trained to help others achieve a high level of self-awareness. Without awareness, there will be no realisation of the challenges someone is experiencing nor willingness to do something about it.

As coaches, we are asking our clients to tell their stories, and then by using powerful questions, paraphrasing, reflecting, and giving feedback, we're able to allow them to look at it all clearly.

This is done without judgment and with a lot of respect. Otherwise, there will be no trust and we won't hear what we need to hear in order to give the right support.

More so, we're empowering our clients, constantly looking at their strengths, finding the positive things, and believing in them (sometimes when they have stopped believing in themselves).

At times, we'll identify a problem of self-love or self-care, and we'll work hard to allow the client to gain confidence in themselves and to practise taking care of themselves.

Now listen: If there's one truth that I learned in my adult life it is that we can only love others to the level at which we love ourselves. No one can care for another if they don't care about themselves. No one can empower another if they don't feel empowered. And no one can allow the growth and development of others if they're not acting themselves from a place of growth mindset.

When I asked my students what is it exactly in the coaching studies that makes them happy to have chosen it, they all, with no hesitation, said that it's the self-development they experience.

As mentioned above, you need to experience a journey of growth and development yourself before you can take another person through such a journey. Good coaching courses will make sure that this is part of what their students experience. The course should give the students ample support as an integrated part by operating an open-door policy, making sure that the availability of the trainer is high, having chat groups and regular student-trainer meetings. I strongly believe that only when someone feels supported that they'll experience learning. Trainers should believe in their students, empower them, and ask them to reflect on their growth daily, weekly, and over the course of time. And ... celebrate every success and achievement.

And guess what? When we celebrate those daily, this becomes a habit of being grateful, and from there, a huge contribution to our happiness.

DIY

We tend to be very critical of ourselves, so there's a helpful coaching exercise in which we ask the client: "What will your best friend say about you?"

Try it. Think about five positive things that your (best) friend can say about you. Look at this list and own it. It's most likely reflecting you at your best self. And if this is challenging, how about asking your friends to write it for you? I bet you're guaranteed to get a lovely list of all the things in you worth celebrating.

To conclude, while it is very important to train yourself in order to become professional coaches, thanks to the fact that coaching is all about people and their development and success, everyone can actually educate themselves on the matter. A foundation course in coaching can be an amazing life skills gift that will help you improve your relationship with almost anyone and will help you in your own amazing growth.

So, get onboard coaching, and let's move your life forward.

ACTIVITY

See the DIY sections within the chapter.

About the Author

Noa Brume is the founder of The International Coaching & Counselling Institute, a European-based training centre for high-performing students and coaches. She is an expert trainer, life coach, and public speaker, bringing over 30 years of experience in teaching people to move their lives forward.

Noa sees training the next generation of confident working coaches as her life mission. She's a great believer in the ability to grow following trauma and spoke about her insights from the time following the death of her newborn son in a TEDx talk, where she shared the importance of helping others as a means to help ourselves.

The unique institute Noa is running brings students from all over the world under one roof, celebrating their diversity and multiculturalism. Students join her coaching courses both in person in The Netherlands and online, as private individuals and via their workplaces.

Email: info@theicci.com
Website: www.theicci.com
Facebook: https://www.facebook.com/TheICCINL
LinkedIn: https://www.linkedin.com/in/noa-brume-mbacp/

CHAPTER 4

The Transformative Power of Shifting Perspectives

By Laurie Cozart, MBA, MCC, MCNLP
CEO and Executive Coach, Positive Psychology
Danville, California

There are things known and there are things unknown, and in between are the doors of perception.

—ALDOUS HUXLEY

When I was six, my brother Ray, who was nine, returned home from school. I was outside playing school teacher, teaching my imaginary class. When I saw Ray, I could tell by his slumped shoulders and the way he walked that he was sad. I wanted to help, but I was only six. I had no tools in my tool kit, so I asked, "What's wrong?" and then just listened.

As my brother talked about his day, his body language changed. He looked lighter. He began to talk faster, and as he described his day and the bullying he had experienced, he seemed relieved, calmer. As his perspective shifted, Ray decided that this was a small moment. He began to look at the situation with a different lens. He had many friends who loved and admired him. I included myself in that group. Both my brothers went out of their way to include me and make me feel special. On this day, I got to return the favor but got so much more. I didn't know this small, meaningful interaction with Ray would become my lifelong passion.

Throughout my career, I noticed what I loved most was supporting the growth and development of others. Years later, I wanted to start my own business, so I started looking for a business mentor. What I found was a coach. I was hooked. I knew this was the career I was meant to pursue. Looking back, I am forever grateful to Ray for being my first coaching client and teaching me the value of exploring situations through multiple lenses.

Coaching conversations are magical places of self-discovery and insight for both coach and client. Within the trust and safety of the coach-client relationship, people will share their worldviews, perspectives, deepest feelings, wishes, hopes, dreams, goals, struggles, and fears. It's a place to work out the complexity of relationships, life, and work. Through the power of listening and inquiry, people are empowered to self-reflect, challenge their thinking, explore new perspectives, and find life-changing solutions.

Self-reflection isn't a natural human instinct. Ryan Holiday says, "The battle for self-awareness is an endless one. The ability to step back and see yourself from a distance, to analyze your flaws and weaknesses, to understand your motivations. This is not only not easy, it's not natural. We were given—cursed with—all sorts of biases and blind spots that work against self-knowledge daily."

Shifting Perspective—Shifts Everything

When considering multiple perspectives, humans often resist because our brain has an addiction to being right. In the 2013 article "Break Your Addiction to Being," author Judith Glaser wrote: "When you argue and win, your brain floods with different hormones: adrenaline and dopamine, which makes you feel good, dominant, even invincible. It's a feeling any of us would want to replicate. So, the next time we're in a tense situation, we fight again. We get addicted to being right."

When working with clients interested in improving their lives, be it relationships, goals, change, or evolving, the most impactful and valuable practice is the ability to support clients through self-reflection and analyzing and shifting their perspectives.

As a coach, I use techniques that get all the senses involved through imagery, metaphor, movement, or kinesthetic exercises, which allow the brain to think differently, create forward momentum, and deepen critical thinking.

Shifting Perspectives: Liz's Story *(adapted from* Coaching Conversations *by Laurie Cozart)*

This exercise or something similar is valuable when supporting individuals to use self-reflection around limiting beliefs or shifting perspective.

Background: In her new role as medical director of a pediatric medical center, Liz guides the care provided and helps define a vision of quality improvement. She is the face of the organization in the community and makes presentations to lawmakers to influence policies that affect children's health. Determined to conquer her fear of public speaking, Liz turned to me for help.

When colleagues describe Liz, they say things like "calm under pressure," "laser-focused in the operating room," and "amazing stamina"—all essential qualities in a top pediatric surgeon. Medical staff also say Liz communicates sensitively with her young patients and their families, and she has a warm sense of humor. It's not hard to see her in the upper echelons of leaders in her field as someone who makes a positive impact on everyone.

That picture of Liz is hard to reconcile with the one she paints of herself when it comes to public speaking:

> Before I even stand up, I work myself into a state of panic—*I can't do this, it's going to be terrible*—so I sound nervous, and the more nervous I sound, the more panicked I get. All the hours I've spent preparing and practicing go out the window, and it's like all my body systems go on high alert. My heart races, my stomach quivers, and I

can't take a full breath. My mind goes blank—suddenly I can't remember what I meant to say, and I trip over simple words. When it comes to being seen and heard, I just shut down.

As she and I had determined what we were here to discuss, I wanted to know when and how Liz started to fear speaking in front of a group. I asked, "What is your first memory of shutting down around being seen and heard?"

Liz had no trouble remembering. She said, "I was about five or six. It was a party for my older brother's birthday, and I was ecstatic because our cousins were there. I was so excited to have girls to play with. We were tearing through the house, shrieking and banging doors. I was leading the way. My father stopped me in my tracks. "Elizabeth! Girls should be seen and not heard! Find something quiet to do."

Liz paused for a moment and then went on. "At first, I was shocked—I had no idea we were doing anything wrong. Then I felt bad, guilty, for displeasing my dad."

I observed, "It sounds like you did an emotional one-eighty, from ecstatic and excited to shocked and guilty."

"Exactly," Liz nodded.

"So looking back as an adult, what are your thoughts around the impact of that experience?"

"I think I've internalized my father's statement about girls not being heard. Even though I know my job requires me to speak up, my overwhelming feeling is doubt, like I shouldn't be doing this. I shouldn't even be in this situation."

"By 'situation,' what do you mean?" I asked.

Liz replied, "Whenever I move into something bigger—more responsibility, more visibility—I feel a sense of 'This is too big for me,' and this memory comes back to me."

Several questions came up for me. I wanted to check any assumptions I might be forming. I repeated the words: "'Girls should be seen and not heard.' Did your father say it often?"

Liz thought for a moment, and then said, "Actually, I can't remember any other time, but believe me, it made an impression!"

"What makes this one time stand out?"

"I don't know. Maybe because I was embarrassed about being scolded in front of my cousins. Maybe because it was so different from the way my dad usually talked to me."

"How did he usually talk to you?"

Liz smiled. "My dad was a doctor. He had an exceptional way of explaining things to me that was kind and patient."

"Besides your feelings when you give a presentation, what evidence do you have that girls—women—shouldn't be heard?" The word "evidence" evoked a change in Liz. One moment, she was back in her childhood, feeling small and uncertain; the next, she was a capable physician, trained in the scientific method.

"I really can't think of anything else—and now that you ask, I'm not even sure I would call what I go through 'evidence.'"

"Tell me more about that."

"Well, for one thing," Liz laughed, "the whole idea that girls shouldn't be heard is ludicrous!"

"What are the chances that your father wasn't serious when he said it?"

Liz smiled and looked past me as if she were remembering something. "It's possible."

Setting the Outcome

At this point, Liz hadn't yet articulated a clear outcome for our session. But we explored enough together to move in that direction. I started with a question: "What would you want your presentations to look like?"

"I want to stop feeling like I'm blowing it."

Liz's response was typical. Most people have a hard time envisioning what they want, so they default to what they don't want. Our job is to help them describe their desired outcome in positive terms.

"You're telling me what you don't want. The question is—what is it you *do* want?"

Liz had recently taken a "360-degree feedback" assessment to understand others' perceptions of her strengths and weaknesses. I asked: "What would you think about starting with your 360 feedback?"

The Transformative Power of Shifting Perspectives

"Okay," Liz said.

"They described you as calm under pressure and laser-focused in the operating room. Some mentioned your amazing stamina. Residents said you communicate sensitively with young patients and their families, and you have a great sense of humor." This is the part of you that's visible to other people. What's happening inside, psychologically?

"I don't know where to start."

Liz thought for a few moments. "Before a surgery, I feel energized. My heart beats a little faster, not because I'm panicked but because I'm looking forward to the work. I've spent most of my life preparing for these hours when I can help someone. When you love what you do, it's not work."

I asked Liz if we could capture her thoughts as we continued. She liked the idea, so I passed her a pad of sticky notes and a black marker.

Here are our questions and answers about performing surgery:

"What kinds of thoughts go through your mind in the operating room?"

She responded, "Things like, 'This is where I belong.'"

"What might make you nervous?" I went on to ask.

"Well, every surgery involves some risk, so I always feel a certain level of tension that keeps me alert. Then there's a percentage of cases where something unexpected happens, and I have literally a few seconds to make a critical decision. That raises my blood pressure."

"So how do you maintain your calm under pressure?"

Liz smiled and explained. "I have a protocol: I say, I am here for situations like this. I've done this perfectly a hundred times. Trust your training. I can see the steps in my mind, even the alternatives if my first plan won't work."

"In the operating room, where is your focus—inward or outward?"

"I'm focusing outward, first on the patient, and then I'm listening to the other doctors and nurses."

I continued, "You've done an amazing job of identifying your beliefs. Who do you believe is responsible to the patient?"

"All of us. I'm part of a surgical team, and we all share the responsibility."

"It sounds like you are at your best in that situation. What are your feelings after a surgery?"

She answered, "I almost always feel deeply satisfied. I know we provided the best possible care."

Liz and I went through a similar line of questioning around her experience speaking and we created a side-by-side view.

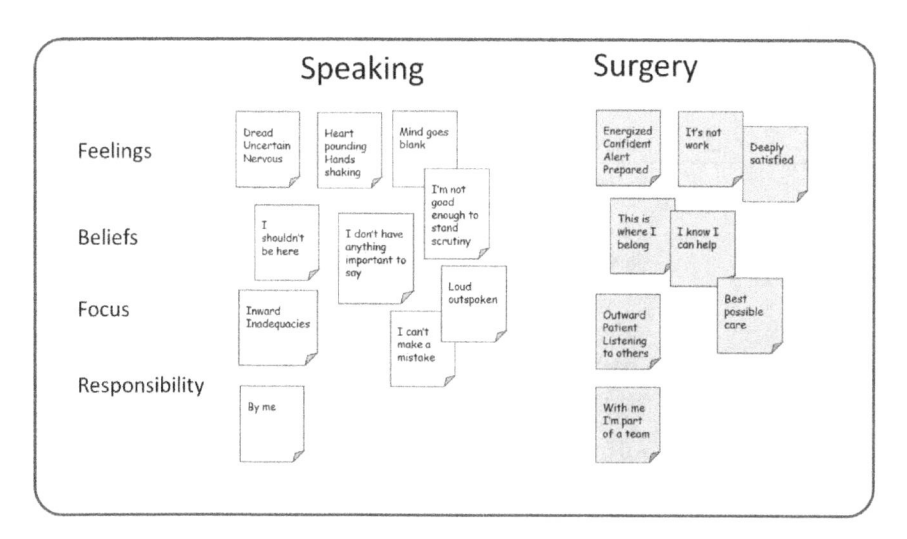

Liz's Current State Graphic

	Speaking	Surgery
Feelings	Dread, Uncertain, Nervous; Heart pounding, Hands shaking; Mind goes blank	Energized, Confident, Alert, Prepared; It's not work; Deeply satisfied
Beliefs	I shouldn't be here; I don't have anything important to say; I'm not good enough to stand scrutiny	This is where I belong; I know I can help
Focus	Inward Inadequacies; I can't make a mistake; Loud outspoken	Outward Patient Listening to others; Best possible care
Responsibility	By me	With me, I'm part of a team

Once Liz had created her comparison graphic, I asked her to stand back from the whiteboard and look at the big picture.

Liz studied the sticky notes for a couple of minutes, and then said, "I'm a completely different person in the operating room. Maybe not from outward appearances but certainly in my inner experience. I've always known my feelings are different. I didn't know that my beliefs about myself are radically different."

"What are your thoughts around that?"

"I thought my problem was my feelings. Now it looks like the bigger issue is what I believe about myself outside the OR, in the role of a leader."

Sensing that Liz had shared enough to describe her desired future state in positive terms, I asked, "The feelings you experience in the operating room, how close would they be to what you want to feel when you give a presentation?"

"Very close. But those two scenarios are like apples and oranges."

"Are they?"

The Transformative Power of Shifting Perspectives

As five silent minutes ticked by, Liz continued to process. Finally, she said, "I can see they're similar enough that I might be able to have some of the same feelings about giving presentations."

Next, Liz created a graphic representation of the outcome she wanted by making a duplicate set of new feelings, beliefs, focus, and responsibility, and sticking them on top of the old. Physically covering up the old with the new symbolized the beginnings of change in Liz's thinking.

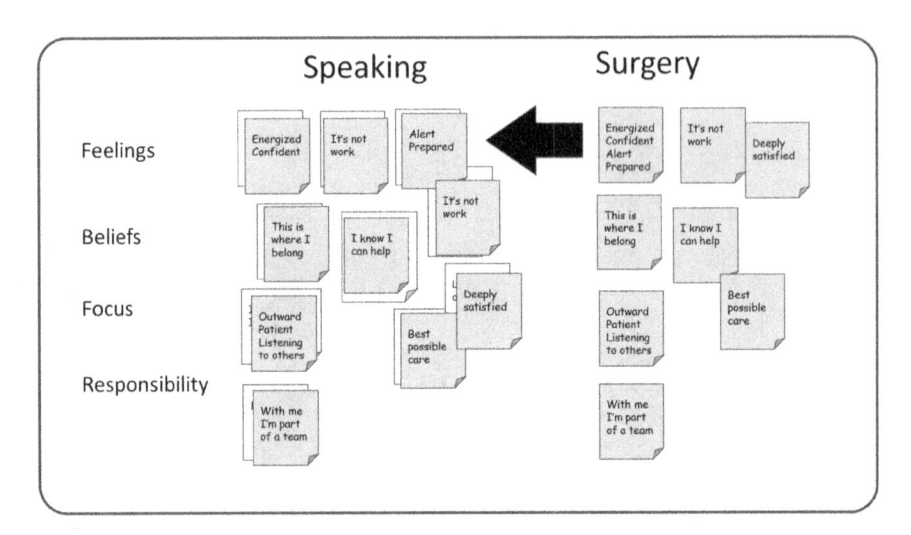

Liz's Future State Graphic

	Speaking	Surgery
Feelings	Energized Confident / It's not work / Alert Prepared	Energized Confident Alert Prepared / It's not work / Deeply satisfied
Beliefs	This is where I belong / I know I can help / It's not work / Deeply satisfied	This is where I belong / I know I can help
Focus	Outward Patient Listening to others / Best possible care	Outward Patient Listening to others / Best possible care
Responsibility	With me I'm part of a team	With me I'm part of a team

Just as clients must choose their perspectives and write their own stories, they must also design their own goals, actions, and accountability measures. Here are some of the questions I asked Liz:

- How do you prepare yourself physically and mentally for surgery? How do you apply that to public speaking?
- What habits support your success?
- What perspectives have shifted?
- How can you carry these new perspectives into your next presentation?
- How will you apply what you've learned about yourself?
- How will you hold yourself accountable for this list?

"The same principle applies to the inevitable setbacks." Liz tells me, "I'm still going to be nervous."

I reminded Liz of how she handles unexpected and critical moments in the operating room.

"You have a protocol for those moments."

"Yes, I do," she said, and then repeated, "*I am here for situations like this. I've done this perfectly a* hundred *times.*"

I pointed to the graphic Liz created, the sticky notes she placed next to the words "Feelings," "Beliefs," "Focus," and "Responsibility."

"What else do you see that you could add to your protocol?"

As we closed out our session, I acknowledged Liz for all the hard work she had done. She left our session with a renewed sense of resolve to become the voice the hospital needed. The following month, Liz gave a keynote at a major fund-raising event. The event resulted in the largest amount of donations ever received at a single event. Liz went on to speak and inspire as the hospital's medical director. Liz also became a sought-after speaker in the medical field, speaking at professional events around the world.

When I think of Liz and when I think back to the conversation with my brother Ray, one of the most important tools I used was so simple: listening. Sometimes the value for the client is just being seen and heard. Remember there is no "one size fits all" technique. We need to remain in full partnership with our clients, with no need to direct or control.

Therefore, I always ask permission and gain agreement before introducing a new technique into the coaching conversation. Taking into consideration the client's preferred learning styles and context.

When we step into every coaching conversation with an openness to travel into another human being's worldview and hold clients capable, the impact can be life-changing.

ACTIVITY

Perceptual Positions

This is a kinesthetic NLP tool that explores different perceptual positions and allows a client to gain new insights into a problem or a challenge, learn more about the dynamics of relationships, and/or learn from an experience. The purpose is to gain wisdom by stepping fully into someone else's shoe and being an objective observer.

Here's what exploring each position offers a client:

Position 1: You

What are your thoughts about your current situation?

Knowing your reality, your thoughts, feelings, beliefs, values, goals, and needs. The first position is essential for a strong sense of knowing yourself and your boundaries.

Position 2: Other

How might others feel about what is happening in this situation?

Others' points of view—how they think, act, and what they value, believe, and feel. The second position is helpful to build empathy and compassion for others.

Position 3: Observer

What do others see? What advice would they give?

The third position helps look at the wider context and consequences for the client and others.

Self, other person, observer.

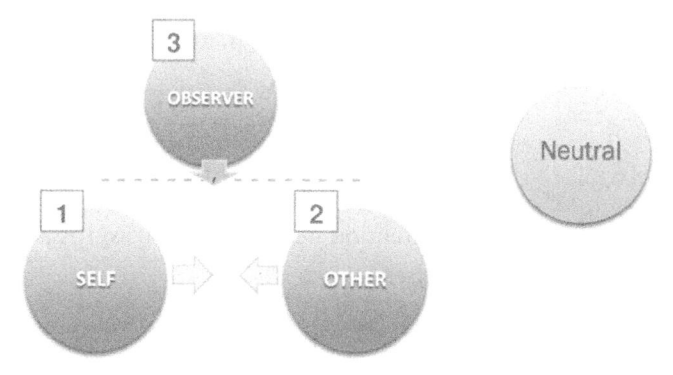

Move to NEUTRAL between each position.

Process:

1. Place cards or objects on the ground identifying three locations for **Self, Other Person**, and **Observer** (as shown in the diagram above). Identify a neutral location apart from the others to which you position the client between each move. Throughout this process, ensure the client uses the word "I" especially when in the **Other Person** position.

2. Ask the client to move to the **Self** position. When fully associated, have the client speak deeply from this position and perspective. Say, "See the situation through your own eyes. Be aware of your thoughts and feelings and how they are impacting the relationship or event."

    - What are your own needs?
    - What do you want to have happen?
    - What else?

Break the client's focus and state, by asking a random question like, "What did you have for lunch?"

3. Now ask the client to move to the **Other Person's** position. When fully associated, ask the client to speak deeply from this position and perspective. Then move them to the neutral position and break state. Imagine what it is like to be the significant other in the situation. Put yourself in their shoes—as if you are looking back at yourself, seeing, hearing, and feeling as the other person would, given their worldview.

   - What are their needs?
   - What do they want to happen?
   - What intention lies behind their words and actions?
   - What else?

Ask the client to break state and move to the Observer position.

4. Move the client to the **Observer** position. With the client disassociated, have them mentally replay the previous exchange between the **Self** and **Other Person** adding their new observations. Ask the client to take a detached viewpoint and look at the whole system or situation from a broader perspective.

   - What do others see when observing the situation?

   Imagine looking at yourself and the other person "over there," seeing the two of them interacting. Pay particular attention to actual behavior, body language, and the sound of their voices.

   - What helpful wisdom or advice would you (or someone else) give yourself seeing things from "over there"?
   - What else is the observer noticing?

Ask the client to move to the neutral position and ask:

- What have you observed?
- What have you learned from this activity?
- What is different/what has changed?
- What new options and choices do you now have?
- How will your insights affect the situation or relationship in the future?
- From what position do you want to work going forward?

Closing

Partner with the client to capture insights and learning by asking open-ended questions that are relevant to the client's outcomes.

- What new perspectives do you need to consider?
- How has your perspective shifted?
- What did you learn about yourself?
- What did you learn about the situation?
- What will you do with this information?
- How would you like to close our session?

Acknowledgment

Acknowledge the client for their work.

About the Author

Laurie Cozart envisions a world where people contribute with confidence and conviction and use their influence in powerful and positive ways. Laurie thinks this is important because every individual has a purpose—that needs to be discovered or uncovered in order to fully contribute to the world. Laurie uses empathy and insight to support clients in building the confidence to step into what's possible.

Laurie is the founder and CEO of Brain Squared Solutions Inc. and is a servant leader in a servant organization. Brain Squared Solutions is dedicated to improving the world by supporting growth in leaders, teams, and organizations so that leaders can create ripple effects of growth and positivity. Her organization serves their clients as consultants, coaches, trainers, facilitators, and strategic partners.

Laurie has been recognized as an accomplished business leader who takes time to connect, build relationships, and support others in finding their voice and fulfilling their goals.

Laurie is a master certified coach (MCC) through the International Coaching Federation and is a master certified NLP coach (MCNLP) who is passionate about bringing coaching into organizations to improve the impact leaders have on teams, organization, families, and communities. She continues to serve on the board of her local ICF chapter and supports the growth of other coaches through coach training, mentor coaching, and coaching supervision. Laurie is the author of *Coaching Conversations: Techniques to Deepen and Broaden the Coaching Experience*, available on Amazon and the soon to be released *Team Coaching Conversations*.

Email: lcozart@brainsquaredsolutions.com
Website: www.brainsquaredsolutions.com
LinkedIn: https://www.linkedin.com/in/lauriecozart/
https://www.linkedin.com/company/brainsquaredsolutions
Facebook: facebook.com/brainsquaredsolutions
Coaching Conversations: https://amzn.to/3sBZsaP

CHAPTER 5

The Heart of Coaching: Active Listening and Assessments

By Sylvie Drapeau
Intuitive Life Coach in Personal Development, Author
Montreal, Quebec, Canada

Above all, be the heroine of your life, not the victim.
—NORA EPHRON

It's crucial for both coaches and clients to have self-discovery materials before starting a coaching program. It's like having a map for your coaching journey. For coaches, it ensures that they can tailor their programs precisely to the client's unique needs, maximizing effectiveness. This approach allows coaches to provide a more personalized and targeted coaching experience, ultimately leading to better outcomes. Equally crucial, it's a service of integrity toward the client. It empowers individuals to embark on a coaching journey fully aligned with their aspirations and challenges, significantly increasing the likelihood of their success in achieving their desired outcomes. It fosters a relationship built on trust and authenticity, creating the ideal foundation for personal growth and transformation.

A Dream Coach and a Dream Client

Now what does it mean to have the perfect client and to be the perfect coach for the client? Well, let's begin by saying that there is no such thing as being perfect. Nothing in this world is perfect, or I'll say it from a different viewpoint. Everyone and everything created in this world is absolutely perfect with all its imperfections.

The perfect life coach for personal development is someone who possesses a deep understanding of personal growth and self-improvement principles. They are empathetic, skilled in active listening, and can guide clients effectively. They've undergone profound personal development themselves and are continually learning and advancing their growth. A perfect life coach should be able to tailor their approach to individual needs on the spot, help clients set and achieve meaningful goals, overcome obstacles, and create a fulfilling and purposeful life. They should also exhibit strong communication, motivation, and problem-solving skills to inspire and support their clients in their journey toward personal development. They're like your friendly guide on your journey to self-improvement.

The ideal personal development client is someone eager for positive change, open to growth, and committed to the coaching process. They embrace their uniqueness, accept feedback, and adjust their self-perception. A perfect client is coachable, curious, and open-minded, understanding their strengths and weaknesses while setting clear goals. They possess self-motivation, self-reflection, patience, resilience, commitment, and accountability. Honesty and integrity are key. Even if a client lacks certain skills but is honest and has integrity, they can embark on a remarkable journey of deep transformation, driven by a fervent desire for change, and open to guidance on how to achieve it.

Coaching these unique clients can be an incredibly transformative experience. They have the potential to inspire you to create innovative coaching programs that challenge your conventional thinking, pushing you to develop fresh teaching strategies, workbooks, and exercises. These clients, marked by their honesty and genuine quest for self-discovery despite their limited self-awareness, can propel you out of your comfort zone as a life coach. This journey can become a roller-coaster ride for your own personal growth, requiring you to recalibrate your own abilities and habits.

In these specific situations, an active coach must activate their sensory system fully. Every sense must be on high alert as you become a keen and attentive listener before you can even embark on guiding a client effectively. It's in these moments that your coaching skills are truly put to the test, leading to significant personal and professional growth.

The Art of Active Listening and Assessments

Becoming an effective active listening coach entails mastering several essential qualities. First and foremost, patience is a cornerstone of this role. To be a successful coach, you must be willing to give your clients the space and time they need to express themselves fully. This patience allows clients to delve into their thoughts and feelings without feeling rushed or interrupted, fostering an environment of trust and openness. Additionally, a profound sense of empathy is vital. As a coach, you must empathize with your clients' experiences, understanding their emotions and perspectives without judgment. This empathy forms a crucial connection that reassures clients that their feelings and concerns are genuinely heard and respected.

Non-verbal communication skills are equally crucial for an active listening coach. Through eye contact, nodding, verbal cues, and body language, you can convey your genuine interest and engagement in the conversation. These cues signal to your clients that you are fully present and focused on their needs. Open-mindedness and curiosity are also key traits to cultivate. You should enter each coaching session with an open mind, ready to explore a client's viewpoints and dig deeper into their thoughts. Encouraging open-ended questions helps a client probe into their thoughts, feelings, and aspirations more profoundly. Furthermore, a commitment to reflection and paraphrasing ensures that you accurately grasp your client's experiences and aids in validating their feelings, which is instrumental in building a trusting coaching relationship. Lastly, respect for your client's thoughts, opinions, and emotions is fundamental in creating a safe, non-judgmental environment that fosters growth and self-discovery. These essential qualities combined with active listening techniques empower coaches to guide their clients effectively toward personal development and success.

In summary, active listening coaches possess qualities that create a nurturing and productive coaching environment, enabling clients to explore their thoughts, emotions, and goals while offering guidance and support. That being said, how does a coach evaluate a client's state of self-awareness, curiosity, open-mindedness, reflectiveness, commitment, receptivity, resiliency, patience, accountability, self-motivation, and honesty?

Initial Assessment of Clients

Evaluating a client's readiness for coaching is a critical step in the process of helping them achieve their personal and professional goals. A skilled life coach begins by conducting an initial assessment. This typically involves having an open and honest conversation with the client to explore their expectations, motivations, and current challenges. Through active listening, the coach gains insights into the client's self-awareness, their willingness to change, and their commitment to the coaching process.

In addition to the initial dialogue, life coaches may use assessment tools like open-ended questions, questionnaires, and quizzes to delve deeper into the client's self-awareness and personal development needs. These tools can help identify areas of strength, areas in need of improvement, and specific goals the client wishes to achieve. As the coaching relationships progress, coaches continuously assess the client's progress, their receptiveness to feedback, and their ability to set and work toward meaningful goals. By carefully evaluating these factors, the life coach tailors their approach to meet the client's unique needs and guide them effectively on their personal or professional development journey. This ongoing assessment ensures that the coaching process remains relevant and impactful throughout the client's growth and transformation.

In early 2002, I was teaching French in an English public high school, serving low-income families and students with behavioral challenges. It was quite a unique role as three certified teachers had left the position previously because of the students' behaviors. I had just returned to my country after six years of traveling, and I applied for the job. I taught students in grades 10, 11, and 12. This high school had an interesting teaching project where students were mixed for extracurricular activities, recess, and lunch, but were separated by gender during class sessions, which I found to be an effective approach for teaching high school teenagers.

In those classes of 36 teenagers, the ones with excellent grades and better behavior were extremely rare, just 2% of the total. Most struggled to focus, lacked interest in learning French, and rarely did their in-class work or homework. At the start of each year, I'd use a workbook I'd created to assess their French knowledge and skills. This assessment helped me group them, always pairing a high performer with lower performers in each group. The high performers stepped into the role of mentoring, guiding, and sharing their understanding and expertise, boosting the confidence and skills of both them and the lower-performing students for all subject-related tasks. This approach aimed to make learning more engaging and effective for everyone.

After creating these groups, it was crucial to clarify the head student mentor's role: sharing knowledge, understanding, experiences, and thought processes to enhance comprehension. As the groups collaborated, it became evident that discordance hindered the learning process. The question emerged: How could these groups work harmoniously? It became evident that for the head student mentors to assist their members effectively, they needed to assess abilities while group members needed to trust in their head mentor's skills and guidance.

This highlights that assessing students or clients doesn't just benefit the coaches or head coaches, as illustrated above, but it's equally valuable for the students or clients themselves who are receiving coaching.

I faced the challenge of finding the right assessment tools to build trust and unveil the abilities between group members and their head student coaches. Open-ended questionnaires and conversations between them were key strategies. I met with the head student coaches to provide assessment tools and guidance, and then I met with the group members to explain the purpose of this new approach, emphasizing that it would create a comfortable and engaging environment for learning, boosting their comprehension and performance. All they needed to do was to become active listeners and apply themselves. Additionally, ongoing feedback and group discussions were introduced to further assess progress and strengthen the coaching process.

In these conversations, it's crucial to share success stories as examples. Emphasize that learning with peers and sharing skills can be as enjoyable as playing sports or watching a friend's cool skateboard tricks. At the start of each class, I introduced a five-minute relaxation exercise, with deep breaths and counting 5, 4, 3, 2, 1 before exhaling. This ritual became so beloved that students even requested it from substitute teachers when I was absent. They found it immensely helpful for improving their focus and overall performance.

You might wonder why, as a life coach, I mention my experience with teenagers. Well, it's because the principles that apply to teenagers are universal. We all seek empowerment, value, appreciation, and support. We have a fundamental need to share our challenges, feelings, and pains with a trusted listener. While many life coaches conduct one-on-one sessions, it's important to remember that effective coaching can take various forms, and one-on-one coaching has proven successful over time. It's about finding the approach that best suits your needs and preferences.

Your one-on-one sessions may be your preferred approach, and it suits your abilities well. However, as life coaches, it's essential not to assume that our coaching style is ideal, even if we are well-versed in personal development. Recently, I reached out to a fellow life coach to discuss a new approach I'm developing and seek her insights. Surprisingly, she declined, claiming she already knew everything about personal development after coaching for over 30 years, believing there was nothing new to learn.

As a life coach, it's important to be confident in your methods and professionalism, but remember that coaching is about the clients, not us. Our role is to assist, guide, and support their self-discovery. While your approach may have worked well for many clients over the years, the field keeps evolving, and it's crucial to adapt your coaching techniques to better suit each individual client's needs. Expertise and success stories should not deter us from embracing new advancements in the field.

Coaching clients in a diverse setting, whether one-on-one or in group, is a vital aspect for all life coaches. Embracing the ever-changing nature of life is essential as everything evolves over time. Coaches should remain open-minded, adapting to the present and welcoming what the future may bring.

Working in groups often benefits clients as it encourages deeper sharing and mutual support. A group of 12 clients is more manageable for a life-coach, allowing the creation of accountability teams that can exchange members every two weeks. This fosters a sense of symbiosis within the group, where clients bond and feel comfortable opening up. The synergy that emerges provides space for self-discovery, empathy, and perspective reframing, empowering clients as they actively aid one another in their personal development journey.

We should actively embrace the changes that the future holds and be part of our clients' success journeys. Our coaching methods, techniques, and tools can evolve to guide them in self-realization. Two vital aspects for raising the likelihood of success are unwavering coaching support, marked by the power of active listening, and a structured assessment process. Including initial and ongoing assessments. Life coaches must adapt to the ever-changing world, from the invention of automobiles to robotics and artificial intelligence, and even cutting-edge surgeries performed through cameras.

Our lifestyle has transformed from handmade bread and hand-washed clothes to today's fast-paced, list-driven lives. Amid this rush, it's crucial for us to understand what we truly need. When a potential client books a call, the key questions are: "How can I best assist this client on their journey? What do they want, and do they truly know themselves? What should I prepare for our first meeting as a life coach?"

Initial Conversation

After a client books a call, we promptly send them a welcoming email along with three different workbook questionnaires or quizzes covering various personal development aspects. These questionnaires or quizzes cover broad categories, aiding clients in pinpointing the specific area of their life they want to focus on. Additionally, they identify any limiting beliefs and daily habits that may be affecting personal development. Their task is to come to the meeting with a one-page summary of their responses, giving them a sense of control and a clear idea of what they want to focus on during our session. This preparation empowers them to engage in the meeting with a strong sense of direction.

The meeting commences with the expected warm welcome and greeting. However, the coach should immediately initiate a conversation, focusing not on the meeting's agenda but on the person. We might comment on their appearance, such as their eyes, or even the artwork in the background. Engaging in small talk about their day, the weather, and other causal topics allows the client to feel comfortable and at ease. This approach transforms the coaching session into a friendly conversation, removing any reservations or discomfort, especially for those who might feel anxious about starting a session with a life coach.

It's essential not to delve into deep questioning right away as this can make the client uncomfortable and defensive. Instead, reassure them that you respect their privacy, and all conversations and materials will remain confidential. Even in the group coaching program, they will be in charge of what they want to share with the group. Let them know that you are a professional, and your discussions are entirely between you and them.

End Initial Conversation

Once you've covered these preliminary aspects, inquire whether they had a chance to complete the workbook questionnaires or quizzes and summarize their answers like asked. If they have, encourage them to share their answers, and for each response, ask them to elaborate their answers or pose questions that will make them elaborate on why it's significant for them. If they haven't finished the questionnaires or quizzes, offer to assist in answering the questions or inquire about their intentions and goals in working with a life coach. We don't blame the client for not completing the tasks we assigned. It provides insights about them, and as their coach, you should observe if it's a recurring habit or a one-time occurrence. If it's a habit, find gentle ways to express your observation and encourage them to make a change, then offer a solution.

Regardless of the situation, during the first call, it's crucial to have the client share their thoughts and experiences while you actively listen. Redirect the conversation to reveal more about their challenges, goals, and the transformation they seek. If possible, conclude the first meeting by providing a strategy to address one of their challenges, particularly those related to limiting beliefs. By offering a solution during this initial 45-minute session, you demonstrate the value of working together and show that they can overcome their obstacles with your guidance, increasing the likelihood of their commitment to the coaching program.

The Heart or Art of Coaching

In summary, active listening coaches possess qualities that create a nurturing and productive coaching environment, enabling clients to explore their thoughts, emotions, and goals while offering guidance and support. Assume that your clients may not know what's best for them until you help them discover their needs and desires. A life coach should not be at the center of the equation but rather in the background, observing, listening, and facilitating clients in finding their own solutions and answers. This approach empowers clients, asserting their self-confidence to manage their situations and challenges, and developing competencies to transform their lives in the way they've always envisioned.

The power of initial and progressive assessments for life coaches lies in their ability to guide and empower clients effectively. Initial assessments provide a starting point, helping clients pinpoint their needs and desires. Progressive assessments, conducted throughout the coaching journey, allow for ongoing self-discovery and personal growth. By using these tools, life coaches create a structured path for clients to identify their challenges, set goals, track progress, and develop tailored strategies for transformation. This approach fosters self-confidence and a sense of control, ultimately leading to successful and meaningful personal development.

ACTIVITY

Becoming an Active Listener— Unlocking Client Transformation

Welcome to the Becoming an Active Listener activity designed to enhance your skills as a life coach. Active listening is a crucial element in your coaching journey, allowing you to build trust, understand your clients deeply, and guide them effectively towards their goals. This activity will help you develop and refine your active listening abilities.

Instructions

1. **Self-Reflection (10 minutes):** Begin by reflecting on your current active listening skills. Consider moments when you felt you were an effective listener and when you might have struggled. Jot down your observations.
2. **Video Observation (30 minutes):** Watch a coaching session on YouTube or journalistic interviews. Use active listening skills. As you watch, focus on the coach's or reporter's active listening skills. Pay attention to their body language, facial expressions, and verbal cues. Identify moments where active listening is evident. Then watch your recorded sessions from previous clients, note, and compare your active listening skills. List which method or techniques you could improve.
3. **Guided Exercises (20 minutes):** Imagine a coaching scenario with a challenging client, or research on YouTube an interview or coaching session you can use. Write down some open-ended questions you would ask to encourage them to open up and share.

Think about active listening skills techniques to write the questions. Develop a hypothetical series of active listening methods and techniques that could have been used.

4. **Role-Play (15 minutes):** Find a colleague or friend willing to participate in a role-play exercise. One of you will take on the role of the coach while the other becomes the client. The coach should practice active listening skills during the conversation, demonstrating empathetic and active listening. Reverse the role-play, so you both practice active listening.

5. **Discussion (10 minutes):** Share your experiences from the role-play exercise with your partner. Discuss what worked well and where there may be room for improvement. Encourage honest feedback.

6. **Goal Setting (10 minutes):** Set specific active listening goals for yourself. These could include maintaining eye contact, using verbal or active cues like, "I hear you," for clients who are auditory learners; "I see what you mean" for visual learners; for kinesthetic learners use face and hand expressions and movement; and for reading/writing learners, show them that you are taking notes. These cues help the coach to avoid interrupting the client and ensure the client that we are still with them, listening and paying attention to their issues.

7. **Practice (15 minutes):** In your next coaching session, consciously apply your active listening goals. Pay attention to your client's words, body language, and emotions. Avoid formulating responses while they're speaking. Instead, focus on truly understanding their perspective.

8. **Reflection (10 minutes):** After your coaching session, take a few minutes to reflect on your performance. Did you meet your active listening goals? What went well, and what could be improved? You may be inclined to watch the recording and analyze it further, taking notes on how and where during the session you could have reacted differently, helping you visualize what and how you can improve next time.

Conclusion

We all know that practice makes perfect, but perfect practice makes it great. Don't be hard on yourself and use your learning style to integrate those techniques. Becoming an active listener is an ongoing process in your coaching journey. By consistently practicing these skills, you'll strengthen your ability to connect with your clients, build trust, and guide them effectively toward their desired transformations. Remember that active listening is a powerful tool that can lead to incredible breakthroughs in your coaching business. Continue to refine your skills and watch your coaching relationships thrive.

About the Author

Sylvie Drapeau is not just a coach; she's a spiritual guide, an intuitive explorer, and a world traveler who hitchhiked for over 15 years. Her lifelong journey into conscious astral projection, which began in her teenage years, paved the way for her mission to empower others in realizing their personal and professional dreams.

Sylvie is the visionary behind *Your Essence of Love*, an online *Self-Love for Success* course, and she has made waves in the personal development world as a co-author of the bestselling book, *The Prosperity Factor*, alongside Joe Vitale.

Sylvie is the CEO of the newly acquired Master Your Life and Ladies Life Designs. Sylvie introduces a ground-breaking coaching program, revolutionizing the landscape of personal development. Her innovative approach centers on developing psychic abilities, leading clients to profound self-discovery, and aligning their life journey with their soul's purpose. With Sylvie, you're not just coached; you're guided on a transformative, soulful expedition to unlock your true potential. LadiesLifeDesigns.com is an online business empowering lady with a ground-breaking soul-driven personal development program.

Website(s): www.SylvieDrapeau.com
www.Your EssenceOf Love.co
www.LadiesLifeDesigns.com

CHAPTER 6

Coaching Tool Kit

By Hope Firsel
Life and Fertility Coach, Rapid Resolution Therapy
Highland Park, Illinois

*Only when we are brave enough to explore the darkness
will we discover the infinite power of our light.*

—Brené Brown

You can overcome anything with a plan and a little hope. With the right mindset, you can navigate any challenge. With the correct mindset, you can triumph over even the most difficult times.

I collaborate with my clients to begin by pinpointing their fears. Often, by discussing their pain, we can deconstruct negative thoughts. Clients must take the time to comprehend the origins of their thoughts, offer themselves compassion, and then start dismantling negativity. I encourage my clients to nurture themselves by practicing self-compassion and understanding. It's crucial for the client to craft their narrative and concentrate on the present moment.

I remind my clients that if they are breathing, they can find gratitude. Many of my clients face infertility, cancer, or divorce—experiences I've personally undergone. I assist my clients in confronting their fears, deciding how they will face them, and then actualizing that vision.

The Process

Below is a suggested outline for the coaching process. However, coaching is an interactive setting where the client drives the agenda.

Phase 1: Initial Overview

Establish the purpose of the coaching experience by creating a brave space where the coach and client quiet the external world and amplify inner voices. Being open and present is an act of courage.

Sample coaching probe: "My intention is for our meetings to provide significant value."

As the client outlines their motivation for seeking a life coach, the coach should listen and utilize this information to define the objectives, opportunities, and processes of the coaching relationship.

Phase 2: Intake Information—Objective

Sample coaching question: "What recent experiences should I know about that can help me assist you?"

Understand the client's perception of their situation, their history, and life perspective to identify potential areas of concern. We need to observe, comprehend why our minds generate certain thoughts, treat them kindly, and let them go. It's time to adopt a new way of thinking.

Where is the client stuck? Where does the belief exist that something shouldn't have occurred? Or where does shame reside?

Phase 3: Dream of the Dream—Subjective— Finding Gratitude in What Is

Encourage the client to articulate their values and future aspirations, and explore all available options. I often introduce meditation and visualization exercises to help the client find inner calmness. Visualization is effective for stress reduction and calming the mind, enhancing the body's equilibrium. After constructing a future vision, help the client understand that by sharing their narrative, they begin to create it.

Coaching tip: Prompt clients to identify things they're grateful for in the present moment. I encourage clients to maintain a gratitude journal, noting at least five things they are thankful for daily.

Phase 4: Self-Discovery/Self-Assessment

The client will consciously define who they want to be when confronting challenges. Existing assumptions, expectations, and self-perceptions will often be reevaluated and redefined. Letting go of emotions is vital for deep relaxation. The coaching conversation should continue to help the client find peace, love, and confidence within.

Coaching probe: "Where in your life are you seeing more ease? Where are you still experiencing triggers?"

Remind the client of all their areas of growth and discipline in this process.

Phase 5: Plan: Create a Short-Term & Long-Term Road Map

The client will formulate short-term strategies to achieve long-term outcomes. The more detailed, the better. Ideally, a daily schedule is employed to outline activities, habits, and a lifestyle that empowers the client to become their best self. Encourage the client and reiterate their success story.

If they are undergoing medical treatment, especially in cases of infertility or cancer, stress management is crucial. Having personally experienced infertility and cancer, I understand the toxic nature of stress. For many, it's a marathon, not a sprint. These clients must learn to separate their mind from their physical body.

Such individuals quickly realize that the mind is their most potent tool. When the body fails or doctors provide discouraging news, the mind remains. They must learn how to calm the mind, converse positively with themselves, and find peace even amid physical discomfort.

Tools

Three-Step Goal Attainment Process (adapted from iPEC)

1. Desire: What do you truly want?
2. Belief: Do you believe you can attain this? Do you believe you deserve it?
3. Acceptance: Believe you already possess what you desire. Embrace your new reality.

A Moment of Mindfulness (*adapted from Eckart Tolle*)

Start sessions with a brief visualization exercise. Guide the client through a centering guided meditation. Ask the client to close their eyes, breathe deeply, and release tension. They envision a chosen color enveloping them, energizing their spirit, and calming their mind. The client's body is eased through this visualization. Once calm, the client contemplates their next thought and then embraces tranquility.

We are often conditioned to believe we are powerless, unable to alter ourselves or our circumstances, or that change is arduous, and life controls us. However, you possess the capacity not just to endure but to emerge from challenges stronger, wiser, and more fulfilled.

Conclude with this: "In this reality, as our body pulses and our mind expands, we have the chance to unite."

Encourage them to maintain a journal, listing their sources of gratitude. Identify moments of miracles. What differed on those days? What's needed to experience such days again?

Encourage a client to compile qualities that embody their vision of an ideal existence. Consider attitudes, beliefs, behaviors, relationships, media consumption, and time utilization.

They can place a childhood photo beside the mirror where they brush their teeth. This practice prompts self-love and care.

Clients should structure their days, incorporating discipline, self-care, rest, and pleasure. Allow clients a five-minute venting session to unload their thoughts.

Set 2 Daily Intentions: What to release? What to manifest?

Daily affirmation: "I possess the free will to choose how I perceive anything or anyone."

My experience with infertility, cancer, and divorce taught me that gratitude can always be found—so long as you're breathing. Your strength exceeds imagination. In darkness, you uncover your true self and what truly matters. Healing need not span years; a few sessions can shift perspectives. Sometimes, a single question or circumstance can connect the mind to new interpretations.

ACTIVITY

Empowerment Questions

Grab a piece of paper and a pen. Now sit in a comfortable position and allow your eyes to close. Breathe in and out, through the mouth, and exhale out the nose to release excess tension. Give yourself a few minutes to go deeper inside. This is your time to leave the stress of the outside world and journey into your inner world to ponder and plan.

1. List your unique gifts that make you come alive. We are all precious beings.
2. Where in your life do you use these characteristics? Consider places, people, and activities.
3. Look at the calendar and schedule these activities consciously into your daily life. Decide where and how you can construct more of those moments within your routine. Mark them down, so you remain accountable and inspired.

About the Author

Hope Lutz Firsel is a women's life coach with extensive expertise in guiding women through life's unexpected challenges. Holding a master's degree in organizational behavior from The London School of Economics and a life coaching certification and training, from iPEC and Rapid Resolution Therapy, she draws wisdom from conquering her traumas. Hope guides women through life's unexpected turns, aiding them in crafting action plans to confront change. Her approach combines strategy, inner child work, and confronting fears. She offers private and group coaching, both online and in-person, blending Eastern and Western philosophies. Her approach empowers clients to chart an effective course through change. Her belief: With a plan and a little hope, any obstacle can be overcome.

Email: hope@hopefirsel.com
Website: www.hopefirsel.com
LinkedIn: Hope Firsel
Facebook: @HopeFirsel
Instagram: @hopefirsel

CHAPTER 7

The Power of Asking a Question

By Curry Glassell
Mentor and Life Coach
Houston, Texas

A question empowers, an answer disempowers.
—Gary Douglas

The most valuable information I've ever received was told to me by my stepfather when I was a young teen.

He said, "Curry, life's too short. Don't take yourself so seriously. Look in the mirror and laugh at yourself as often as possible." His advice has become a true gift and a blessing as a parent and a life coach. Working with people who have so many "serious problems," whether it is a death in the family, money, relationships, all the drama. What if instead of a melodrama, our life was more of a comedy? Would that be a little easier? For me, that was a big yes. I was a single mom of two little boys, and I was looking for parenting tools to alleviate my drama in my life.

Not to say that my clients' problems aren't important. I am in this field to inspire, assist, and facilitate people around their problems and to make their lives better. My philosophy includes assisting them to add a little laughter and less significance to their big problems. As Mary Poppins reminds us, "Just a spoonful of sugar makes the medicine go down."

If I were asked, "What is the most important thing you can do to give value to your clients?" I would say, "Teach them how to ask a question."

Does that sound simple?

Learning to Ask Questions

Many, many years ago, Gary Douglas said to me, "The question empowers, the answer disempowers." I've found that asking questions has been a very successful tool thus far. I've used it with myself, with my clients, as well as when assisting my children. Only after I was able to empower myself did I choose to become a life coach and, therefore, branched out to work with others.

In terms of my formal education through my college degree, it seemed that the goal was to be "right," and if I was not "right" according to their program, then I was "wrong." Have you had a similar experience?

Looking back, I realize that I was taught in school to "look for the answer" that the teacher wanted or that the test required.

I, as well as many other people, grew up looking for answers and looking for how to be right and not wrong. It was scary to ask a question in school because if I was wrong, I would be shamed. For many people, this fear, unconsciously, continues into adulthood.

Do you remember when you were in school and asked a question, sometimes the teachers got really annoyed? That's when many kids stop asking questions. Did you? If kids were not discouraged from asking questions, it would allow them to flourish at school. Point is: These children grow into adults who now don't ask questions and are now your clients. Once I recognized this, teaching my kids to ask questions became very important. Hopefully, if my kids ever go to a life coach, they'll have a jumpstart.

Learning to ask a question was like—WOW. It blew me away at first.

Asking a question changed the energy. Why? Because it allowed me to perceive and recognize that there were many more options than right or wrong.

Although simple, it took me some time and practice to learn this "new" concept and apply it to my daily life.

Sometimes there was no specific question; there was just an energy that was bothersome.

How do you address an energy? A thought, a feeling, an emotion? It became obvious that asking a question could even address the energies that are not specific or logical.

Raising my kids was my greatest practice to begin to ask questions.

For instance, I would sit with my children while they were doing their homework. What I found out is that sometimes asking them a question made them very angry because they wanted me to do their homework for them. They would ask me questions and I would ask them questions in response instead of giving them an answer.

"Where can you find the answer to that math problem? Is it in the front of the book? In the middle of the book? Or in the back of the book?"

They would ponder those questions. It took a little practice and eventually they would figure it out.

This is like teaching your kids and your client's magic.

In the long run, my listening and asking them questions caused them to grow and learn how to manage their own homework and eventually their own life challenges.

What had occurred for me also started to occur for my kids and my clients. In turn, this showed me that it was much more empowering to ask them a question than to tell them what I thought about their situation.

I desire to empower and inspire my clients to trust themselves, and that begins with them learning how to ask questions and listen for their own knowledge of the issue. When you begin to ask questions, closed questions as well as open-ended questions, it allows your client to have the space to look at their life from a larger point of view.

For example, in parenting, which is almost like coaching, as I incorporated questions into my daily life raising my boys, I began to look at how to empower them and their issues as they grew up. My life with my boys began to be more exciting and more empowering for all of us.

Another question I suggested to my children when they could not decide what class or what sport to play was, "What would your year be like if you chose that? What will that create for you and your year at school? And your next year?"

Another question could be, "What would occur if you chose that sport? What would occur if you chose that other sport?" which are both questions to get an awareness. Asking, "Should I do this or should I do that?" is more about "What is the 'right' choice?" from logic, which is not awareness.

Can you sense the difference? I suggest removing all the shoulds anyway. Try it out. See if you like it and if it works for you.

Asking for What's Right Instead of What's Wrong

Another great question I have used, which has totally transformed my life is, "What is right about me?" instead of the very popular go-to question, "What is wrong with me?"

Consider asking, "What's right about me? What's right about me? What's right about the situation that I may not be getting?" and giving those questions some room to breathe.

There's a gift and a greatness in everything people choose to encounter in their lives. Asking someone a question that shifts their perspective out of being wrong can be life-changing.

So basically, this is about learning how to ask a question instead of automatically going into a conclusion or answer.

So if something didn't go "right" in my life, instead of getting mad at myself or judging myself, I would say, "Well, okay, what's right about this that I'm not getting yet?"

Asking a question will open up different doors and will empower you and, therefore, also empower your client.

I've worked with lots of people over the past 20 years and what I found is that as a life coach, most people want you to provide direction or give them an answer. Basically, they want you to fix their life and they also get to blame you if your advice doesn't work out.

The key to getting around this is to teach the client to ask questions themselves. This is true empowerment of the client and one of the greatest gifts you can share with anyone.

So it's more like a dance to teach a client how to ask a question instead of giving them an answer. That's facilitation. There is a movement.

One of my teachers, Jean Houston, would say, "If you are stuck on a subject, stand up and walk or dance around for one to three minutes to get the energy in motion and moving through you and your body." Asking a question basically does the same thing on an energetic level; it stimulates movement.

Another teacher of mine, Gary Douglas, in reference to my son who was acting out in school and had "way too much" energy for the classroom, suggested that he ask the teacher: "Could I go out into the hall and do some jumping jacks and then return shortly?" When he did this, the teacher agreed, and they all had a much easier time for the rest of the year. Most importantly, my son didn't fail that year and didn't feel wrong about his enthusiasm and abundance of energy. It changed my son's whole experience at school.

Asking About Your Client's Knowing

When you begin to work with someone, a great way to empower your client's knowing and awareness is to simply ask them. It's also easier for the coach. For example, you can ask, "Well, what do you know about this?"

First of all, why is this easier for the coach? If I don't have to come up with solutions and/or answers for a client, then I mainly have to hone my listening skills. Then I can ask them questions that will direct them into looking at their particular point of view about their problems. This leads to more possible questions and more openings for the client to gather information about their own awareness. The client then discovers there is more than one solution. What do they know? What would be best for them?

Because my basic point of view is that the person who is my client really, truly knows what is best for them. This is absolutely about honoring and acknowledging the client.

I have begun to see very clearly the importance of honoring the other person's choice, even though you don't agree with it or you don't like it, that doesn't matter at all. It's the other person's choice. When you honor their choice and you ask them questions about it, you give them a chance to see if the choice is still working for them.

Have they come to you because their choice is not working for them? Yes?

Then your job becomes listening and leading them to discover their own solutions and possibilities.

So, you are training yourself to become a listener, a leader, and I would say, a positive manipulator.

Asking a question to yourself empowers you to look at what you know. Asking a question to your client empowers your client to look at what they know.

Asking questions is a completely different way of living and looking at your life.

Asking About the Future

Here's a great example of using a question in my daily life that occurred recently. I was looking to rent a condo in Florida to be near my eldest son and his wife who were very close to having their second baby.

If I'm going to come to Florida, I would like to see the sea and the sky and feel my feet in the sand every day. That was my desire. That was my dream. My son, who is a realtor, sent me a list of seven places.

"Am I gonna do this logically or energetically? What would be a question that could help me choose? What would be an easy question? What would contribute to my life and my future?" Question, question, question …

So I skimmed over the properties he sent and asked: "So which one of you would contribute to my future the most?" And I just looked over them and one of the photos of properties just stood out. I opened up that one property and looked at all the details. That was it. That one had everything that I wanted in a condo and it was on the beach.

So then I called my son and I said, "Can you find out about this one?" He put a call into a leasing agent and reported back that he was going to meet him at the condo in half an hour and would give me a call from there. We had a FaceTime call and sealed the deal within two hours.

That just made my life and my move so easy. That's what a question can do. It can make your life easier.

Closed and Open Questions

One specific way to begin with a "closed" question is to invite your client to answer with a yes or no response. For instance, as simple as "Is your name … [blank] …? Is your job … [blank] …? Is your hair color … [blank] …?" It is a bit like learning to muscle test but not exactly; it's getting to know your own response muscle.

This is a basic way to begin to listen to energies and sense them because they are very, very subtle, like a whisper or like the wind, and it can take quite a bit of practice to build this muscle. In this case, "Practice makes perfect" is true. This is very much like learning to become your own guru.

An open-ended question example would be asking your client, "Where and when did you go against your own knowing in the past?" For example, "Did you ever eat something that caused you to be sick?" or "Did you ever sleep with someone that you knew you shouldn't have?"

Ask them to give you examples. Educating your client to perceive and acknowledge when they made a choice to go against their own knowledge is invaluable.

Asking for Something in Particular

I'll give you one more example from parenting because this also works for anyone.

When my boys were very little, they were often shy to ask a question or didn't realize they could ask a question. So, I said to them, "Hey, guys, let me tell you something important. If you ask me for something you desire, like ice cream, what's going to happen? What are the chances of you getting a yes and what are your chances of you getting a no? 50/50!"

I went on to point out, "If you don't ask me the question, if you don't ask me for the ice cream, what is the chance of you getting what you'd like? Zero percent. It's pretty obvious, right? This is true for any desire you will ever have."

So don't stop yourself from asking because there's always a 50% chance you'll get a yes.

And don't be upset if you get a no; just keep asking.

In Summary

This tool is about learning to ask a question for yourself and your client. If you do not ask a question, there is no possibility for the person or our universe to respond to you or to open a door for you. This is the value of asking for something with a question. Learning how to ask a question and learning how to empower yourself and others leads to not just surviving this life but actually thriving and empowering your clients to thrive as well.

So now, how do you ask your client a question that's empowering to them? Well, you must become a great listener. This is the key.

Become the best listener in the world, become such a great listener that you can repeat exactly what your client says back to them. And with that, with those tools in hand, you'll be able to create a very valuable business.

Alright, good luck.

ACTIVITY

Questioning Practice

Questions to Practice Your Yes/No Response

- "Is your name … [blank] …?"
- "Is your job … [blank] …?"
- "Is your hair color … [blank] …?"

Open Up to Get Awareness

- "What would occur if I chose this?"
- "What would my life be like if I chose that?"
- "What will that create for me and my year at [place or organization] and my next year?"
- "What am I actually asking for?"

Access Your Knowing

- "What do I know about this?"
- "What do I actually already know about this?"

Get Out of Feeling Wrong about Yourself or About a Situation

- "What's right about me?"
- "What's right about the situation that I may not be getting?"

Getting Clear What the Options Are and What Choices Will Work for You

- "What are the options? Which option would contribute to my future the most"
- "What would be a question that could help me choose?"

"Take 10 and Be with It"—An Exercise to Assist Coaches and Their Clients to Relax and Receive Information

This is a quick meditation for life coaches. If you are feeling upset, angry, or frustrated with something or someone, count to ten (maybe 20) before you respond or take action. Sometimes, if it's an upsetting email, take 24 hours before you respond. Then, to become present with the situation, your question, or your problem, do this:

- Allow a slow breath in, count—1, 2, 3, 4, 5—hold—1, 2, 3, 4, 5—and breathe out with another 1, 2, 3, 4, 5 counts. Breathing out helps to relax your nervous system.
- Begin with counting to ten slowly.
- Let your awareness sink down to the gut level of your body.
- Observe: Where in your body are you feeling or sensing the upset, anger, or frustration?

No matter how negative or intense the situation may be for you, keep breathing and relaxing through it and ask these questions:

- "What is the power in this …?"
- "What is the gift in this …?"

No answer required. You are looking for awareness. Let the questions shift the energy and open another possibility for you.

About the Author

Curry Glassell is a producer, author, speaker, philanthropist, and art-loving mother of two. She always seeks to promote her personal mission, which is to help others experience profound joy in their adult lives by shifting habitual thinking, so they can make more satisfying choices in the future.

Born to be a glamorous globetrotter, raised in oil patch opulence, educated in New York City, and finished with a big dose of reality as a struggling single mom. In her mid-forties, Curry pivoted and took total charge of her own life to forge a courageous new path—supercharged with a desire to create more conscious change and personal empowerment for herself and others.

Email: info@curryglassell.com
Website: www.curryglassell.com
Socials
Instagram: @curryglassell https://www.instagram.com/CurryGlassell
Facebook: https://www.facebook.com/CurryGlassellCF
Youtube: https://www.youtube.com/@curryglasselllifecoach

CHAPTER 8

The Power of Knowing— Spiritual Coaching with Psychedelics

By Magdalena Haver
Spiritual Life Coach, Psychedelic Guide & Facilitator
Amsterdam, The Netherlands

One way to think about psychedelics is that they can help you get out of your own way and see things as they actually are, not as you think they are.

—MICHAEL POLLAN

In the following chapter, I'll share my journey to becoming a spiritual and psychedelic coach, offering insights and considerations for those intrigued by this unique path.

You have to do it on your own, but you don't have to do it alone.

This has been my own motto that beautifully captures the essence of what I believe people seek in coaching. They want to be heard, witnessed, seen, and supported. Asked deep questions, while allowing their personal journey to unfold and understanding to grow. My story is based on years of experiences with clients who managed to transform in a way I had never witnessed before.

I hadn't initially envisioned myself as a coach. During a phase when my life seemed to be lacking direction, terms like "life purpose" and "exploration of consciousness" started showing up to me. At that point, while navigating a challenging personal journey, I was travelling across the globe, seeking guidance and healing from mentors and teachers.

It was during this quest that spiritual coaching found me. I went through intensive training, cleared my exams, organised a studio, and began working with the first clients.

What Is "Spiritual Coaching"?

Spiritual coaching is for those who are seeking to connect with themselves on a deeper level. It is based on traditional life coaching and integrates spirituality into the sessions. It combines inner process, intuition, and subconscious with action skills and seeks connection through mind, heart, and gut. The idea behind it is to help people find their way by following their true, unconditioned self, free from any limitations created by conditioning and ego.

Things were progressing well, but a pivotal moment arose when I incorporated psychedelics into my work.

Already before I opened my coaching practice, psychedelics and plant medicine had made a profound impact on my life. It was my therapist, skilled in navigating altered states of consciousness, who first introduced me to this realm. During a particularly tough period for me, he suggested a psychedelic session, which opened a door to a new dimension of exploration of consciousness.

Since then, working with these substances has been the most transformative self-work I have ever undertaken. My fascination for their immense healing potential has continuously grown, and I immersed myself in various psychedelic experiences that became sources of a profound calling.

What Are Psychedelics?

Psychedelics are substances that primarily induce non-ordinary states of consciousness. They can alter what we normally see, hear, and feel, often leading to what's commonly known as a "trip." Some of the most well-known examples of psychedelics include mescaline, LSD, psilocybin, and DMT.

Scientific research, as illustrated by MRI scans, has shown the formation of new neural pathways and brain connections when using psychedelics. These new pathways can shift our perspective, enabling us to transcend our ego, as well as familial, societal, or religious conditioning—what I often refer to as "the shoulds."

There is substantial historical evidence indicating that our ancestors knew about the special powers of certain plants and fungi and were using them since the earliest times. In Europe, Albert Hofmann's synthesis of LSD in 1938 started an exploration of these compounds to be later suppressed due to societal and political shifts in the '60s. Now, led by passionate supporters and scientists, we are living what is called a psychedelic renaissance.

Psychedelics are usually known to be used for therapy. There is now strong evidence that they can also support those in search of personal growth and transformation, who want to connect to their life purpose, enhance creativity, make shifts in career, personal relations, or move certain blockages. This is where coaching can play a powerful role.

When I started coaching with psychedelics, my approach was primarily intuitive. I worked with psilocybin containing truffles—compounds that are legal in the Netherlands. Psilocybin is known for increasing connections, developing creativity and self-awareness, and having a deep impact on perception of life.

I undertook intense practitioner's training, gaining necessary knowledge in areas such as participant screening, understanding contraindications, the importance of preparation and integration, ethics, knowledge of the basis of trauma, and somatic work.

I was also working for a big international organization facilitating group retreats— this hands-on experience, combined with the training has provided me with the knowledge and confidence to work with clients on a one-on-one basis.

How Do We Know That We Are Truly Ready to Become a Psychedelic Coach?

How do we know when we've learned enough, especially when dealing with something as sensitive as altered states? One thing became clear to me: "You learn best by doing." Taking first steps needed a lot of guts, honesty, and diving deep into self-understanding. It wasn't easy, and I faced my own challenges. At the same time, nothing has ever felt so right—the transformation I was seeing in my clients was mind-blowing. I received some great testimonials, words of appreciation, and gratitude. It helped me to keep going, exploring, and daring.

Selecting Your Approach and Choosing the Right Substance

As a psychedelic coach, you will find a multitude of pathways to engage with this work. Your role may involve guiding clients through the entirety of their psychedelic journey, including preparation and integration. Alternatively, you might specialize in microdosing coaching or focus on preparing and integrating clients before and after experiences conducted elsewhere.

There is a huge variety of psychedelics and plant medicine, and you need to assess yourself which substances you will work with. Your choice will depend on personal experience, training, and comfort level. From how I see it, you can only go as far with a client as to how far you have gone yourself. This includes establishing a profound connection with your chosen medicine and staying open to its intuitive messages.

Just as importantly, always consider the legal implications in your region. In most countries, psychedelics are not legal. Some places permit specific compounds for religious practices, while others have decriminalised their possession and use, reducing or eliminating penalties.

In the Netherlands where I live and work, the use of so-called "magic truffles" is legal, and they can be safely and openly incorporated into coaching sessions and therapy. Psilocybin, their active ingredient, is not considered addictive as it does not induce drug-seeking behaviour or physical dependence. Psilocybin offers mainly an inner journey, and for most of the time, your client will appear to be in a dream-like state. While pre- and post-session talks are vital, there is usually a minimum intervention during the journey itself.

MDMA and ketamine are wonderfully proven successful in therapy but work usually under a clinical setting or underground. MDMA is very relational and there is talking, physical contact, and interaction. Ketamine journeys are short but can greatly deepen insights and access territories of the psyche that are usually hidden.

Other substances like mescaline cacti are usually used in indigenous people's territories under ritualistic and shamanic contexts. The famous mother of the plants—Ayahuasca—is extremely popular in Central and South America, as well as DMT and 5MeODMT, available in certain decriminalised settings or underground. All these substances demand a very careful selection of knowledgeable and experienced guides.

As a psychedelic coach, you will probably not be able to work with most of these compounds, but you may help prepare clients to choose a retreat that is in a region where their use is legal or decriminalised.

What Qualities Are Essential for a Psychedelic Coach?

Two words come to mind: courage and integrity. I would invite you to ask yourself what integrity means to you, define your values, and write your own mission statement and code of ethics.

Drafting your personal mission statement will crystalise your prevailing values and vision. Establishing a clear ethical code is not only essential for client transparency but also serves as your own personal compass. Ethics, especially within the realm of psychedelic facilitation, can greatly help guide you through non-conventional dynamics, as the altered states present unique challenges and considerations often absent in traditional coaching or therapy.

There are some considerations specific for psychedelic work. An example can be a prevalent pitfall from psychedelic facilitators and coaches, and that is over eagerness to help. Through experience, I've learned the power of the principle: "Let the client be," placing trust in their own innate healing capacities. Interference should be minimal and intuitive. As coaches, we know how essential it is to refrain from comments, opinions, or advice. In a psychedelic context, it becomes even more important as individuals can be very suggestible and open.

We need to be mindful to prioritise our own healing and well-being; self-care is essential. Regular supervision and peer consultations offer opportunities to share both triumphs and challenges.

It is also vital to recognise and accept your own limitations. Whenever necessary, do not hesitate to refer clients to other specialists. Maintaining a ready list of trusted therapists is a wise practice.

What Are Essential Parts of Work with Psychedelics?

Preparation—it starts from your initial contact with a client and a crucial part of it is screening. That means assessing whether a person is ready, qualified, if it is safe for them to work with the psychedelic substances, and whether we, as their guide, feel comfortable.

A start is creating a form that will already ask a few most important questions and eliminate common contraindications. We can ask about previous experiences with similar substances, history of trauma, and more. After clearing the form, we can assess further readiness via direct contact with an introduction call. During this process, risks need to always be taken into consideration, and clients should be encouraged to consult medical professionals if needed.

Building relationships will establish trust—you can do it by conducting more coaching sessions prior to the psychedelic journey during which you will discuss various aspects of life, including identifying limiting beliefs and obstacles preventing a client from moving forward.

Practical preparation is necessary for both the guide and the client. Central to this is the well-known "set and setting" concept—mindset and environment significantly influence each psychedelic experience. Several tips can help prepare the right mindset. These may include dietary considerations, slowing down, meditation, connecting with nature, self-observation, and journaling. It's also advisable to distance from substances like alcohol, individuals, or energies that might be negative, as well as violent media.

The "setting" refers to the location of the psychedelic journey. Key elements are comfort, safety, appropriate music, and temperature. Authenticity is essential in this space. While psychedelic work can be done in various settings and there aren't definitive guidelines, I always aim to create a warm ambiance with candles, pleasant aromas, fresh flowers, and soft blankets. Often, I invite clients to bring meaningful objects or photos that might support their journey.

Selection of the right music is crucial. There are numerous playlists tailored for psilocybin journeys; it is often recommended to choose music either without lyrics or with lyrics in an unfamiliar language. Music serves as a grounding anchor for clients, especially during challenging experiences. I customise the music selection, but having a universal playlist is also an option.

Setting an intention is key. Intentions address specific life themes and set direction. As part of the preparation process, I help a client refine their intention. I send a form with supportive questions, and we usually dedicate a separate session to focus on intention setting.

Coach's Personal Preparation and Self-care

Before initiating any psychedelic session, I ensure I am well-rested, centred, and grounded. Prior to the session, I usually review notes from coaching and preparatory discussions and have participants sign a consent form. Every psychedelic coach and practitioner should be equipped with an emergency protocol, ensuring they are prepared for any unlikely events. This includes undergoing a first aid course and understanding typical situations that may arise, along with recognising when further assistance is necessary.

Commonly Asked Questions During the Preparation Process

In my experience, three inquiries frequently arise: "What if I experience a challenging trip?" and "Will I remember the experience?" Additionally, clients often inquire about achieving ego dissolution.

To answer the first question, I usually recall a famous saying that under a right set and setting, there are no bad trips; there might be challenging trips. Bad trips typically occur in unsuitable environments, like clubs or when mixed with alcohol or other substances. This can lead to confusion or panic. However, in the proper environment with adequate preparation, the risk of a bad trip diminishes greatly. During a conscious, intentional journey, a client may face confrontations, but these can result in growth and progress. Embracing the mantra "what you resist persists" can help. I advise a client to stay open and curious, wondering, "what is this teaching me?" and set a reminder: "this, too shall pass." Often, knowing that they are not alone and are supported and guided is enough for a client to feel safe.

One key to a good experience is the art of letting go. Surrendering to the process, rather than resisting, can make a difference. Preparing for the unknown requires humility and trust.

Concerning remembering important messages: Once, during my own journey, I was downloading insights that I really wanted to remember. The message I received was that "my heart will remember." The therapeutic transformations that occur during psychedelic experiences can remain with us beyond the confines of the conscious mind. Naturally, many insights will still be retained. A guide can play a pivotal role here by documenting any revelations a client might share during or after the journey.

Ego dissolution is a term made popular by recent documentaries and refers to the experience of losing the sense of self or personal identity. It is important to set a client's expectation that this phenomenon does not always happen, and even if so, it can take different forms.

Integration

The integration process is vital after each psychedelic experience and can beautifully bridge into following coaching sessions. As a coach, your role is to facilitate a reflection, probing with open-ended questions, encouraging the client to articulate their experiences in terms of images, insights, and memories from the journey. Explore any shifts in their pattern recognition, heightened awareness, and the changes they're inclined to make in their life. Encourage them to identify self-assigned tasks that align with their insights. At its core, integration seeks to ground the individual, helping them derive meaning from their experience.

Microdosing

Another widely embraced method of coaching with psychedelics is microdosing. It involves consuming minimal amounts of a psychedelic substance a few times a week over several weeks. I have created a detailed microdosing guide that I share with my clients before initiating the process, informing them about potential benefits, risks, and ethical considerations. I place emphasis on the importance of setting intentions. I also help them to integrate insights into their daily life and connect to broader microdosing and psychedelic communities.

In Summary

There are many levels of approaching this work. Despite millennia of use, adequate research is still lacking to craft definitive guides on the safest and most effective use of psychedelic substances. Our understanding of this realm is largely based on experiential knowledge, and it's not without risks. Pursuing this path demands courage, integrity, humility, trust, and a strong professional network and support system.

Not all coaches, and not every client, are prepared to embark on this profound journey. However, for those who do venture forth, the rewards are remarkable. Coaching with psychedelics can usher clients towards transformative outcomes: getting to know themselves at the deepest level, embracing surrender, fostering vulnerability, aligning with life's purpose, and cultivating deeper emotions.

Psychedelic coaching goes beyond simple work; it becomes a life of service where we deeply connect with the mystery of existence. This journey bears immense responsibility, necessitating the delicate balance of self-care, continuous personal growth, humility, trust, and a commitment to authenticity. Our role is not to perform but to remain non-judgmental, harmonising knowledge with intuition, and creating a nurturing space for both our client and ourselves.

I wish for everyone reading this to experience a depth of love and satisfaction similar to what I have encountered through my work. I envision a future where psychedelic substances gain wider acceptance and legality, and utilised with reverence and responsibility, causing no harm but instead radiating love and compassion. May they assist people in reaching their utmost potential, aligning with their authentic self and purpose, and contributing to a better world.

ACTIVITY

Preparation and Integration with Psychedelics

The following are some preparation and integration tips and questions you may use to bridge a client's psychedelic experience with your coaching sessions.

I. Preparation: intentional mental and emotional work done in anticipation of a psychedelic experience

1. Start painting a picture of the client's life, discerning their goals, desires, limiting beliefs, and blockages. You may use a discovery session formula.
2. Connect a client's goals to intentions: "What do I want to change/focus on/transform?" or "How do I explain my intention to a five-year-old?"
3. Connect to values: "What do I value in my life?"
4. Ask them to visualise their future self above fears and beliefs: "What kind of person do I need to be to realise those goals/dreams/intentions?"
5. Connect to a bigger vision: "Why does this matter to me?"

II. **Integration:** incorporating insights and lessons gained from a psychedelic experience into one's daily life for personal growth and well-being.

1. Create a special atmosphere, recall smells, or play music that was used during a psychedelic session or retreat your client went to.

2. Ask one question at a time and give space. Remember how vulnerable psychedelic experiences can be and that it takes longer to put feelings into words. Ask open versus closed questions. Examples:

- "How was the experience for you?"
- "What are you celebrating or concluding?"
- "Reflecting on your original intentions, how did the experience align?"
- "What lessons or insights emerged from the session?"
- "How will you integrate the lessons into daily life?"
- "What additional support might enhance the benefits of your experience?"

About the Author

Magdalena Haver is a psychedelic practitioner and certified life and spiritual coach who blends spirituality with pragmatic insights. Born and raised in Poland, she travelled globally and connected with teachers and mentors, nurturing her experiential learning and inner transformation.

After following practical teachings and wisdom traditions, Magdalena discovered a passion for psychedelics that opened gates to more understanding, love, and compassion. She has engaged with multiple substances and is continuously learning from her own medicine journeys with both indigenous and Western guides.

Magdalena works from her studio in central Amsterdam and online, guiding individuals and groups to connect with who they truly are and cultivating trust as a core guidance towards inner knowing.

With experience in event organization and management, she also curates group retreats that align with her deepest passions.

Magdalina is a co-parent to two grown children and a beloved golden retriever. She is empathetic, intuitive, and caring.

Email: herosjourneycoach@gmail.com
Website: https://herosjourneycoach.com
Socials: https://www.instagram.com/herosjourneycoach/
https://www.facebook.com/HerosJourneySpiritualCoaching/

CHAPTER 9

Achieving Goals with the Power of the Five Whys

By Alissa Janey
Author, Life Coach, Creator of ElevateRadiate.com
Minneapolis, Minnesota

If I had an hour to solve a problem, I'd spend 55 minutes thinking about the problem and five minutes thinking about solutions.

—Einstein

Consider a time when a client was working toward a goal, and despite their best efforts, they weren't progressing as quickly as they had hoped. Perhaps it was because they were concentrating on the symptoms rather than the underlying problem. Whatever the reason, it can be hard for some people to determine what roadblocks are keeping them from reaching their goal. And that's where a personal life coach can help.

Life coaches serve as guiding beacons, illuminating the path toward self-discovery and meaningful change. They are the architects of transformation, helping individuals clarify their goals and navigate the landscapes of their deepest motivations, desires, and aspirations. One of the ways life coaches achieve this is by employing an array of tools and techniques, each designed to uncover hidden potential and pave the way for a more fulfilling existence.

Among these tools exists a remarkably simple yet highly impactful method that has the power to reveal the root causes of challenges, surface meaningful insights, and facilitate lasting transformation. This method, known as the "Five Whys," is more than just a problem-solving technique; it is a profound lens through which life coaches can help their clients gain unparalleled insights and identify those hidden roadblocks. The Five Whys technique involves asking your client "why" five times. Each sequential "why" question probes deeper under the layers that contribute to a specific goal or challenge. Doing so helps uncover the primary motivations and experiences that influence an individual's perspective and why they might be getting stuck.

Whether you're a first-time life coach or experienced and hoping to expand your tool kit, the Five Whys offers a framework to guide your client toward transformation. This technique sparks a journey of self-discovery, growth, and empowerment guided by the belief that beneath every dream, goal, or challenge lies an opportunity for us to learn more about our inner, authentic self.

So let's begin this adventure together and see how the Five Whys technique can be used in the world of life coaching. We'll unlock the door to a future brimming with possibility and purpose.

The Origin of the Five Whys Technique and How It Works

The Five Whys approach to problem-solving originated from the Toyota Production System, a production philosophy created by the Japanese automaker Toyota. The technique is used in lean manufacturing and process optimization to address issues of quality and efficiency. Even though this method was originally designed for the manufacturing industry, it can be applied to any aspect of life—specifically useful in goal achievement.

The Five Whys is a structured and iterative approach to problem solving. To begin the process, start with a goal or specific issue. Each "why" builds upon the previous answer, allowing you to uncover new insights and connections. By the time you reach the final "why," you will likely have peeled back the surface layers of a problem and identified the underlying motivations for a specific goal or obstacles preventing your client from moving forward.

When used in coaching, this, in turn, leads to a more comprehensive understanding that allows for targeted solutions and a higher level of follow-through and commitment from clients to achieve their goals—because they have clarity on precisely "why" a specific goal is important to them.

Exploring the Motivations Behind Our Goals

The Five Whys is a powerful method of discovering the underlying motivations that result from our distinct experiences, thoughts, and emotions. As we progressively ask, "Why?" we're prompted to tune in to our inner self and access the wisdom within to explore the reason behind our goals. Once we tap into this knowledge, we have a clearer understanding of what truly fuels our aspirations. In the end, the Five Whys serve as our compass, leading us straight to our heart's deepest desires and motivations and helping us reconnect with our authentic self.

Let's look at an example between a life coach and their client of how the Five Whys can reveal a client's internal motivations in a coaching session.

Goal: Gabriella wants to open a successful Italian restaurant business.

1st Why: Why do you want to open an Italian restaurant? I want to open an Italian restaurant because I am passionate about making Italian food and want to share my family recipes with the community.

2nd Why: Why do you have a passion for cooking Italian food and want to share your family recipes with your community? I have a passion for cooking Italian food because it's something I would do for free the rest of my life. It also reminds me of wonderful childhood memories cooking with my grandmother. Additionally, when I create food that people enjoy, I feel a sense of accomplishment and fulfillment.

3rd Why: Why do memories with your grandmother and making food that people enjoy create a desire to open an Italian restaurant? Some of my best childhood memories are cooking with my grandmother. We spent quality time bonding and creating memories filled with laughter and joy. I would love the opportunity to recreate those moments.

I also want to spend more time doing activities that I'm passionate about, such as cooking and running a business, because my current job does not align with my strengths or passions.

4th Why: Why is it important for you to recreate these memories by opening an Italian restaurant? I want to provide a place where people can go with their family and friends to make their own special memories and spend quality time together.

5th Why: Why is it important for you to create a place where friends and family can spend quality time together? At this point in my life, I want to focus on what my purpose and legacy could be. After self-reflecting, I realized that one of my key priorities is to make a positive impact in people's lives. I find fulfillment and purpose when I contribute to the world in a way that brings people together.

Five Whys Process Internal Motivation Findings

Through the Five Whys method, Gabriella lit up when sharing her reasons for wanting to open a restaurant. Gabriella's driving force behind her goal appears to be intrinsic motivation with the desire to relive positive childhood memories, promote internal fulfillment and purpose, and contribute to a happier and more connected community. Her findings act as a building block to inform business decisions pertaining to branding, customer engagement, restaurant offerings, and atmosphere.

Revealing Hidden Obstacles

The Five Whys technique can be extremely effective at disclosing concealed obstacles that may be impeding a client's progress toward their goals. Recognizing these obstacles aids in the ability to develop targeted strategies for overcoming them and make meaningful progress toward a client's aspirations. Because with each sequential "why," we peel back the surface to expose the primary causes of potential setbacks, uncovering barriers that may otherwise remain unidentified.

For example, if your client's goal is to advance in their career but they feel stuck in a specific position, the Five Whys could reveal that a skill or experience gap is preventing them from advancing.

Here's another example that demonstrates how a life coach can use the Five Whys to help Michael get to the root of why he may not be advancing to a manager-level job.

Issue: Michael aspires to advance into a manager-level position in his career. He has applied for manager positions but hasn't received any offers.

1st Why: Why haven't you received a job offer for manager positions you've applied for? Human resources shared that my resume doesn't highlight leadership or team management experience.

2nd Why: Why doesn't your resume include leadership and team management experience? My supervisor hasn't delegated team management or leadership responsibilities to me even though I consistently meet performance expectations.

3rd Why: Why do you think your supervisor hasn't delegated team management responsibilities to you? I haven't had a career development conversation about my future career goals and aspirations with my supervisor.

4th Why: Why haven't you had a career development conversation with your supervisor? My touch-base meetings with my supervisor primarily focus on business updates rather than personal growth or future career aspirations.

5th Why: Why don't you and your manager discuss your career aspirations and development? I guess neither one of us has ever brought it up.

What's the root cause preventing Michael from securing a manager position?

The Five Whys analysis makes it apparent that a lack of proven leadership and team management experience are holding him back from advancing to a manager position. Michael also has not shared his career goals with his supervisor, which could be preventing his supervisor from considering Michael for new projects that would help him gain relevant skills and experiences.

Potential solutions for Michael include:

- Seeking leadership opportunities on his current team, such as leading initiatives and mentoring less-experienced team members
- Discussing with his supervisor that his career aspirations are to gain leadership responsibilities and advance to a managerial position
- Exploring lateral moves that offer an opportunity to lead cross-functional projects and gain exposure in other divisions
- Pursuing training programs or certifications to close any skill gaps

The Five Whys method brought Michael's barriers to the surface for him to observe, process, and create a plan to begin tackling. By discussing his career aspirations with his manager, developing a career development plan, and making progress against this plan, Michael should have a solid strategy to advance into a manager position.

Tips for Building Rapport to Create an Open and Trusting Environment

The essence of the Five Whys can help your clients discover the origin of challenges and explore their thoughts and emotions on a deeper level, leading to valuable insight. Therefore, it is essential to create a space where clients feel safe opening up.

Establishing rapport with your client throughout the coaching process, respecting their boundaries, and maintaining client confidentiality aids in laying a solid foundation for productive and supportive coaching relationships. When coaches build a connection and sense of trust, a safe and nonjudgmental space can be created where clients feel comfortable to freely share their thoughts, struggles, and aspirations.

Here are a few strategies that life coaches can use to establish rapport with clients:

1. **Find common ground.** The more sincere interest you show in your client, the more likely they will relax and open up. Use open-ended questions to discover high-level details about your client, such as where they grew up, their favorite sport, a recent movie they've seen, or a conference they've attended.
2. **Promote active listening.** Active listening involves creating an environment in which your client feels heard, understood, and supported. Practice active listening by providing your full attention, maintaining eye contact, and using such verbal cues as "I understand" and "Tell me more." Let your clients see that you empathize with their experience, even if you haven't personally gone through the exact same situation.
3. **Acknowledge progress.** Incorporating genuine and specific feedback about the client's progress can have a significant impact on building and maintaining rapport. Celebrate the client's progress and achievements, no matter how big or small.

Overall, a strong rapport leads to more effective coaching that encompasses an open environment, invaluable discoveries, and—ultimately—stronger client outcomes.

The Five Whys Approach with Clients

Life coaches can use the Five Whys in many ways to help clients explore their goals and challenges. In addition, remember that every person is unique and has their own set of experiences, circumstances, and outcomes they want to achieve; therefore, customizing your approach to each client is key. Outlined below is a high-level approach to use as a starting point.

The Five Whys Approach

Step 1: Begin with the goal or issue. To begin the Five Whys process, ask the client to clearly articulate their goal. Their objective could be related to personal development, their career, or another aspect of life. If applicable, you want your client to share what they believe may be preventing them from achieving their goal.

Step 2: Introduce the Five Whys. Explain the Five Whys technique to the client and share that the objective is to listen for their underlying motivations, obstacles, and emotions associated with their goal. Emphasize that the process works best when they have an open mind and sincere introspection.

Step 3: Start with the first "why." Ask your client why they want to achieve their specific goal or why they believe a particular issue is occurring. This initiates the questioning process and the beginning of understanding their motivation or obstacle. For example, if the client's issue is procrastination on training for a marathon, ask them why they believe they're procrastinating.

Step 4: Repeat and dig further. As you continue through the process, ask your client "why" in response to each one of their answers. Be sure to give them time to process their thoughts, emotions, and answers. After their initial response, ask "why" again to get to the heart of their reasons. Repeat this process to uncover deeper layers of motivation, obstacles, and potential fears.

For example: "Why are you working overtime at your job instead of spending time on self-care and training for the marathon?"

Step 5: Identify and summarize key findings. As you continue through the "why" iterations, you and your client will likely get closer to understanding the motivations behind their goal, any core issues, or a belief that could be causing the issue. You may even discover that they're lacking a particular skill, experience, or mindset that would help them move closer to their goal.

Next, help your client summarize any insights you've gained from the Five Whys process.

Action Planning Following the Five Whys Process

Following the Five Whys approach, use the ideas below to facilitate the action planning process with your client.

1. Create a SMART goal and develop an action plan. Based on insights gathered from the Five Whys approach, work with your client to clearly articulate their goal and create a detailed action plan.

This plan should include specific steps, strategies, and resources to achieve the goal, shift their perspective, and make a plan to overcome obstacles.

The SMART goal method is one way to achieve this. SMART goals provide a simple and effective framework to organize an action plan. By setting SMART goals, you can help your client focus on their priorities, track their progress, and celebrate achievement along the way.

SMART goals:

Specific
Measurable
Achievable
Relevant
Timely

For SMART goal tools and examples, reference ElevateRadiate.com.

2. Make a commitment. Referencing your client's SMART goal and action plan, have your client create an "I will ..." statement that will help them progress toward their goal.

3. Conduct regular check-in meetings. Schedule regular sessions with your client to review the progress they've made against their commitments, make any necessary adjustments, and provide support as needed.

4. Adapt and evolve when necessary. Goals, dreams, and motivations can change over time. Be open to revisiting the Five Whys process as needed—especially if your client's circumstances or aspirations evolve.

As we conclude this chapter on the Five Whys technique, it's clear that this method is more than just a problem-solving tool. It's a gateway to unlocking a client's core motivations and obstacles keeping them from achieving their objectives.

Remember Gabriella, who through the Five Whys discovered that her motivation to open an Italian restaurant stretched beyond the strictly business-related—it was about reconnecting with cherished memories and giving back to her community. It's a reminder that your client's goals aren't just about what they want to achieve but why.

The Five Whys technique also illuminates hidden obstacles, like what we saw from Michael's career aspirations. And once these challenges are brought to the forefront, you can create targeted strategies to tackle them.

But the true power is not just in the technique itself; it's in the relationship you build with your clients. Focus on creating a safe, trusting space where they can open up and share their thoughts and dreams.

The techniques in this chapter will help your client understand their true aspirations, flush out obstacles holding them back, and most importantly help them focus their time and energy on the right goals. These breakthroughs can reignite a spark within your client to move forward with enthusiasm, hope, and confidence.

For more on the Five Ways process or my other coaching tools, visit ElevateRadiate.com.

ACTIVITY

The Five Whys

Instructions: Use the Five Whys to help your client get to the root of their problem or understand the underlying motivation behind their goal. Once your client defines their goal on a surface level, ask your client "why" five times until you get to your final answer. Reference the Five Why approach outlined in this chapter for additional support.

Five Whys Exercise Template	Five Whys Exercise (Example)
1) Starting goal: _____.	1) Starting goal: <u>I want to lose weight</u>.
2) Ask the Five Whys: • 1st Why: • 2nd Why: • 3rd Why: • 4th Why: • 5th Why: 3) Refine your goal:	2) Ask the Five Whys: • 1st Why: I need to lose weight. • 2nd Why: I want to be healthier. • 3rd Why: I would like to live a long and healthy life. • 4th Why: When I am older, I hope to be strong and healthy enough to do the things I love such as yoga, traveling, and watching my future grandchildren. • 5th Why: Living a high-quality life is important to me. I also want to make good memories with the people I love. 3) **Refine your goal:** To live a long, high-quality life, so I can do the things I love when I am older such as yoga, travel, and create memories with the people that I love.

About the Author

Alissa Janey is a life coach, blogger, author, and the creator of ElevateRadiate.com. Elevate Radiate is an online coaching platform that helps people tap into their own inner strength to live a more intentional life and realize their dreams and goals.

Alissa has 20 years of corporate experience with Fortune 500 companies where she led initiatives in goal setting, coaching, change management, career development, performance and talent management, and culture training. She is a certified change facilitator and has won several awards for her work.

Check out Alissa's website, other books, and free tools here:

- Website and blog: www.ElevateRadiate.com
- Free Living Intentional Planning Guide and other tools: www.ElevateRadiate.com and go to Self-Paced Tools
- Career Development Guide: www.ElevateRadiate.com/shop
- Self-Love Journal: www.ElevateRadiate.com/shop

Follow Alissa on social media to receive weekly inspirational messages and videos at Elevate Radiate by Alissa Janey.

Email: ElevateRadiatebyAlissa@gmail.com
LinkedIn: Alissa Janey
Facebook: Elevate Radiate by Alissa Janey
Pinterest: Elevate Radiate by Alissa
Instagram: Elevate Radiate by Alissa Janey

CHAPTER 10

Meet Me in the Middle: Inner Alignment as Free Medicine

By Miranda Jol (BSc: Joy of Life)
Owner, Magnetic Vibes; Life Coach
Amersfoort, Netherlands

> *You were never broken.*
> —Jeff Foster

How a 12-year-old and four Matruschka dolls brought back the memory of the essence of our being: a blueprint for connecting to our true self, others, and the world.

How It All Started

The telephone rang. I picked up the phone. An affected, emotional voice came from the other end: "Do you also coach children"? For a moment, I was confused. I could clearly sense that something was very wrong by the way the man on the other end of the line sounded. I listened with my most present attention.

"Can you tell me who you are and what's going on?" I asked.

A stressed voice said, "I'm sorry if I may be bothering you, but it's important. My name is Andrew and you coached me a while ago in a business situation. There is a serious situation involving my 12-year-old son Jonathan."

I now recognized the voice and heard myself say, "Yes, I remember. And, yes, I do coach souls, independent of their age." A deep sigh sounded on the other end of the line.

I invited him to share what was bothering him so much. He started to talk, stumbling over his words.

His son was suspended from school. He had stabbed another boy with scissors. As a supreme defense mechanism in a situation where he was being bullied. There was a lot of commotion among the students, the parents, and the boys involved. There was shame, fear, anger, grief. Not exactly easy emotions to connect with within ourselves.

I was listening and could see and understand that the father, and everyone involved, was clearly upset and looking for ways to handle this. It was clear that he felt his son should take responsibility for what he had done. That it was not okay to stab someone.

And he felt angry and powerless because his son had done this in response to bullying. Behavior that is quite common among children. And also not a desired behavior.

And from certain expressions I could tell that it also affected the father himself. Standing up for yourself, setting a boundary without showing aggression.

I felt immediately that several questions were intertwined. The most important question had to be addressed first: How did we invite an 12-year-old boy to open up and restore the connection within himself, the situation with school, and the other boys? Not exactly easy questions.

And the feeling of urgency to find an opening within this difficult situation.

And I knew, the only moment we really have in life is in the now.

From life and coaching experience, it was clear to me I was not asked for a format, a solution, a system, or a conviction. The only thing I really had to do was to be there, curious, with an open mind, not knowing where it would lead, and to trust.

At that time, I couldn't have known that this case would completely turn the way I worked in my practice upside down.

The next morning, a timid, sad-looking boy reluctantly entered my practice. Jonathan looked at me, assuming that I would be yet another adult who condemned his act. He hardly dared to look at me. I saw eyes filled with shame and felt a heart full of sadness. I realised then that the special thing about being in the presence of children is that they purely show what something is. I welcomed him and realised that I didn't mean to make small talk with him.

The most direct path to liberation from whatever was trapped was to speak and invite the truth from the heart. Mine and his. So I started and told him that his father had called me and asked for my guidance in the situation that happened the day before at school. Furthermore, I told him shortly what I did for work in my coaching practice.

I asked him how he felt that morning.

"Bad, tired, scared, and angry" were the first words that came to his mind. He nodded when I said that wasn't a nice place to be.

I asked how he felt at my office. He was strikingly present in the moment.

He looked around and then said softly, "It feels relaxed here, and I'm a little nervous." He told me everyone was so angry or disappointed in him that he did not know what to do anymore. Next to that, he was suspended from school, and he couldn't help but think about the situation all the time. It was like a movie repeating itself over and over.

He said he found it very difficult to talk about it. I asked him if it was okay to find a way with me to talk about it.

He said to me, "I feel okay to talk with you." And with frightened eyes, he added, "But I don't know how … and I'm afraid to tell what happened."

I asked him how that was for him, and he answered, "I feel like I am in a prison in my head. And I don't know how to get out of that prison."

When I asked where he felt all that in his body, he was surprisingly precise: a heavy feeling in his head, shortness of breath, a tight throat, a stabbing feeling near his heart.

As he said this, he looked at me with tearful eyes. It touched me. I felt the sadness and powerlessness, and I told him that. Exactly so.

There was silence, and I let it be. That moment still stands out today.

He then looked at me and said with his eyes cast down and emotion in his voice, "But I don't know what to do."

Speaking my truth in that moment, I answered, "I don't know yet at the moment. Shall we find that out together?"

A sigh escaped him, and he looked at me, a little brighter.

That's Where the Magic Came In

At this point, I'll explain how an unexpected tool guided us to step into an energy field and unveil the key to turn around this situation to a perspective of growth.

It felt like there was a little more space now. I invited him to look around and asked him if there were any objects in my practice that might help him tell the story. He briefly looked around and was very clear about his choice: "The dolls ... that fit together in different sizes," he said. They were actually the Matruschka dolls that I had intuitively purchased a few weeks before.

I asked him to take the four dolls apart and asked him what he thought the dolls stood for in the situation that had taken place at school.

First of all, we decided together what each figure symbolized. He explained the smallest puppet was him as a new born baby, free, happy, and unprejudiced. He told me that part was still somewhere in him. He didn't have access to it at that moment. As a second doll, he took the largest one. And told me that it represented who he was now. At the age of 12.

He described that it felt like he was a volcano. Which had erupted the day before. When I asked how that felt, he said he literally felt bloated, and something inside him snapped.

At that moment, it was visible how incredibly sincere he showed what was happening inside him. His clarity and ability to convey what was going on was striking. I carefully explored whether he was ready to tell what happened the day before. At that moment in the conversation, I experienced that it arose in the moment, as if we were being guided.

For a moment, the scared look appeared in his eyes again, but then he opened up.

The day before, he had a task in the kitchen of his school. At some point, a few of his classmates came in, and as often happened, they started to tease him. He felt awkward and unsafe in the small space because he had nowhere to go. At some point, he wanted to leave the room, and one of the boys blocked his way and made fun of him in the process. At that point, something snapped; there were scissors within his reach and he lashed out with them. Not to harm the specific boy but to get away.

As he told this, there were tears in his eyes. "I didn't mean to hurt him, but I was so fed up with it ... and didn't know how to stop it. I know what I did was wrong and I deeply regret it."

He continued, "And I am angry too. Because it feels unfair. I was doing an assignment in the kitchen, and they came in there for no reason. Just to make fun of me. I reacted in the wrong way, which I shouldn't have done. I'm the only one not allowed to go to school now. I have to have all kinds of difficult conversations, and they get off scot-free."

Then unexpectedly, he takes the second smallest doll, and the conversation takes a different turn.

"When I was 7 years old, I was allowed to help my father in his shop; I liked that very much. And was very proud of my father who had built it all up himself. Until one day, a customer was very rude to my father and didn't want to pay for something he had worked really hard for. I felt how unfair this was, and that made me feel so angry and sad. I wished I could do something about that to help him. At that moment, my father didn't say anything, but when something happened at home, he would explode. That's what I was afraid of. I don't really know how else to do that either. So that's where the second smallest doll is standing for. I hold back because I don't know what to do."

I complimented him on how he managed to put that into words and then asked him what the third figure stood for.

Without hesitation, he then placed the four figures in a row and explained, "The smallest doll represents the relaxed state, like a baby. Free to laugh, cry, sleep, move, etc. The second figure does a step back; it shows how I adapt under stress. I clam up and no longer know what to say. And the third figure represents the way I decided how to deal with it."

"'And how would that be?' I asked him in the flow of his view.

"Oh, for now I feel I need to become strong, not show that I am afraid. Afraid of being alone. All by myself in this situation." And he moved the third puppet a step forward, so the puppets were no longer in a row.

There was now a long silence. I saw that Jonathan was completely absorbed in the story of what the puppets stood for. He spoke in a very vulnerable and truthful manner and had momentarily forgotten what the situation was like the previous day. I asked him what the biggest puppet represented, and he said that it represented everything he is now.

"Yesterday, I felt like a tense slingshot and now more like a slack rope. In any case, wobbly."

It was very special to observe how he simply and truthfully described what was happening inside him and what the puppets stood for.

He also showed me that when all the figures within him were in one line, he felt okay. And that wasn't the feeling now. There were two breaks in the line. The first fault line was where the second puppet stepped back, and the second one where the third puppet decided to be/do/pretend something he really wasn't.

From that perspective, I could ask him questions about what he thought was needed in this situation and what could be of help to him. We talked from the position of several puppets about apologizing, talking to his parents and teacher about this, and about how he felt about going back to school.

Gradually, I saw a 12-year-old boy bounce back into a healthy line and show remorse and ownership. And a special clear wisdom. Even a smile because he felt like he had some new ideas on how to do this from now on.

That afternoon, I worked with the same "'Matruschka Method" with his parents. It turned out that they also recognized patterns within themselves, and they also saw ways to approach this differently in themselves. Step out of the drama triangle and child decisions in their own lives.

To step into an infinite field of energy that is always there to provide.

And easily return/reset to their own alignment by the magic of imagining how to put their four Matruschka dolls in a solid line. From where it feels easy, relaxed, open, connected, free to speak, to set boundaries, to show vulnerability, to ask for help.

After and during these conversations with Jonathan and his parents, I realized this could be a simple tool. To magically self-regulate situations and emotions to inner peace. Where the alignment of soul, heart, body, and mind magically allow the situation to work out in a way the mind never could have.

Miranda Jol (BSc: Joy of Life)

The Matruschka Method ®

To align and meet yourself in the middle

Soul blueprint	Child conclusion(s)	Survival Strategies	Self-image in the now
(Birth)	(0-11 years)	(12-25 years)	(repeat pattern/ free flow)
Aligned	1st fault line	2nd fault line	assumed identity

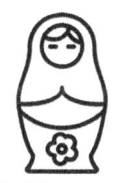

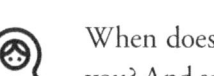

When does it fit your soul? Check with one question: Is it for you? And so, it feels relaxed, excited, gives energy, goosebumps, joy, flow!

What happened in this period (0–11) that caused a fault line? What did you conclude as a child? (Default conclusions as: I'm not good enough, I have to work hard, or I don't belong here.) How did you hold back? Where do you still feel that in your body?

Which behavior did you develop in this period (12–25) to survive/thrive? Fight, flight, freeze, fear, work hard, perfectionism, rationalism, emotional manipulation, addiction to …, etc.

What is your "favorite problem" in your life now? How does that show up as a red line in your life? What does the pattern look like every time? What would your life look and feel like when you are totally free as you are naturally from within?

ACTIVITY

An Embodiment Exercise to Align the Matruschka Dolls in Yourself and Experience Inner Freedom

Being present to your whole inner world = Your own free medicine

Invite yourself or another person to:
Close your eyes and focus inside, from head to toe. Breathe slowly, and be present with what is. Be and stay with whatever there is with all the attention of all your body cells.

Think about a child decision you made and the place it is stored in your body.

Give space with your breath to the whole spectrum of feelings around the child decision in your body.

Let your breath follow its own stream.

Listen to what your body tells you. It's so smart, your real brain.

Ask your body where it's stored and if you can allow all your cells to that feeling.

Listen, feel, listen, feel … breathe.

With two feet on the floor, eyes closed, and attention to your heart, bring the energy to your gut. Decide to let it go, whatever the story is. Give the energy back to where it belongs: Source.

Fill your whole body by taking a breath. Fill your whole body with a stream of light and love. Ask your body to show you the way, and let things work out.

All is energy. Trust that your light body and connection with Source will automatically reset itself. Ask for help from Source to reset your cells on your soul's blueprint. Give yourself in that moment what you think you need from others. If you let it go, you get the flow!

About the Author

She not only had a gift to offer the world, she had a gift to offer to herself. Maybe it didn't matter so much if the world held it. Maybe what mattered was that she did.

Miranda Jol was born and raised in a working-class family in a small village in the Netherlands. As a young child, she knew how to manifest things effortlessly and miraculously. During life, she learned beliefs, university education, and programming, which stood in the way of this gift. At least, that's what she thought. Through all kinds of life experiences, travelling and working with amazing and wise people and projects in the world, she learned that we can create our life all by ourselves. In alignment with an infinite energy field, in that, she experienced great freedom and pleasure.

In her own company Magnetics (2001), she brings her soul mission to the world—fanning the fire from the source that we are: unconditional love. She feels grateful to be a source of inspiration and connection for so many world souls. She remembers people to the freedom that they are and have from within so that they can live a soulful, healthy, inspired, and connected life.

Email: magnetics@ziggo.nl
Website: www.magneticvibes.nl
LinkedIn: www.linkedin.com/in/MirandaJol

CHAPTER 11

The Transformational Guide to Flourishing Personally and Professionally

By Zelda Okia, MD
Life and Weight Loss Coach, Forensic Pathologist
Milwaukee, Wisconsin

In today's fast-paced world where life pulses at the speed of technology, as an entrepreneur and business owner, it's hard not to get caught up in the demands of owning a business as you chase after the elusive success that others appear to find easily.

I remember nights when my husband, Patrick, would awaken in the wee hours of the morning and find me in our spare bedroom staring into the screen of my laptop or fitfully typing away with the faint blue hue of the computer casting long shadows across the room. I was building what I thought was our dream business of the future. But I was not thinking about the cost. How can you count the cost when you never even imagine that there is one?

Entrepreneurship, for all its allure, can be a very intoxicating maze. There's always more to do. There are always more places to go and always more people to meet and more to achieve. Just the sweet aroma of success is enough to keep you buried away in the energy and intoxication of creation. But again, at what cost?

Amidst the chaos, you may discover all too late that among the many rewards of all your efforts, you have also secretly, yet devastatingly created a tattered marriage, a growing distance from your children, a dependence on a little too much alcohol, a growing waistline, or an unexpected and untimely negative health diagnosis, growing within the shadows of too many missed doctor's appointments.

I remember the day that my hubby called me during one of my one-on-one discovery coffee chats, telling me that he was not doing well and I needed to come home immediately. I remember thinking, "Why now?" and feeling a growing irritation as I thought it wasn't the time for his drama. After all, wasn't it his idea that I quit my job and go full-time into this entrepreneurship journey?

On our 45-minute drive to the Veterans Administration Hospital, my husband gave me an earful of many nights of sleeplessness, loneliness, and perceived abandonment, while I spent hours shut away in the spare bedroom that had become my office. It was during that drive that I came to realize how much my hubby and our marriage together really meant to me. And how at risk I was of losing all of it to pursue this fledgling enterprise that was nowhere near being able to support us. But this realization and my hubby's candor, vulnerability, and honesty set us both on track to discovering a magic wand that has not only sustained us and our marriage but has served to continuously propel us forward. That magic wand—transformational self-care.

Through this process, we discovered a tool that helps us to see our value through the lens of self-care. Self-care is a tool for greater productivity, efficiency, and achievement of many of our goals. We now offer these transformational tools to our clients in our Self-Care 101 Masterclass. It is our hope in this brief book chapter to share how transformational self-care not only changed our lives for the better but also to show you how it can absolutely change your life and bring greater depth and meaning into your business, propelling you forward to levels of unimaginable success.

The Four Tools of Transformational Self-Care: Self-Awareness, Work-Life Balance, Thought Work, and Emotional Mastery

Tool One: Self-Awareness

Entrepreneurship can often feel like riding a treadmill with a gradually increasing incline and faster pace. Yet many of us entrepreneurs never realize that we are the ones completely in charge of that pace. Many like myself are on a non-stop quest to find the newest and best gadget or surprise to wow our current or prospective clients. While others are stuck playing a numbers game of who has the fastest hustle.

However, when you realize that your most precious resource isn't capital or connections, but time, that sets a new light on priorities. When you consider the 80/20 rule and sit down to analyze which 80% of your hustle or business is producing only 20% of your results, you start to really consider your priorities.

One of the tools that we introduce to our clients is a trademarked personality profile test. Once you complete the quick assessment in 90 seconds or less, you very soon realize that it isn't just a tool to mirror who you are. Rather, it serves as a guiding strategy, directing you toward what truly matters. It assists in aligning your tasks with your core values, priorities, and strengths, determining that the pivotal 20% of your effort is invested in areas leveraging your innate skills and expertise.

This tool allows you to align your daily schedule of activities with your priorities and your areas of expertise. Imagine working "on" your job, shaping it, designing it, and crafting it into an extension of who you are and how you wish to express yourself in the world.

How might things change when you approach your work from this perspective? Knowing what matters most to you, this tool can aid you to not only know yourself better. But you are also able to share it with co-workers, family, friends, and associates, and create better relationships both professionally and personally.

Tool Two: Achieving Harmony in Work and Life

You have likely been asked at some point along your entrepreneurial journey, "How do you balance it all?" You may shy away from the question or suppress that rising feeling of imposter syndrome. But the honest truth? You don't.

What if the operating word isn't "balance" but "harmony"? The Webster's dictionary's definition of "harmonize" is "a pleasing arrangement of parts or congruence." The life wheel exercise is your guide in revealing the areas of your life that may need some attention. Life balance or congruence is not about creating equal slices of an overwhelmed or overfilled pie but ensuring that each slice is as fulfilling as the other while recognizing that smaller slices do not necessarily equate to less importance.

I may make the conscious decision to make less money on one project in favor of another which may bring me more fulfillment in the moment. Additionally, attending my child's sporting event may make more sense than spending that extra hour in the office.

Mental resilience in business isn't necessarily about avoiding stress. It's about managing it. When you're at peace with all facets of your life, challenges in business become puzzles to solve or work through rather than heavy burdens to drag around as an unwanted weight. It is developing life harmony through stimulating creativity rather than causing burnout.

Tool 3: Thought Work—The Thought Cycle: Your Business Strategy's Secret Weapon

Let's start this section with a definition of the thought cycle. Every decision we make in business stems from a chain reaction of thoughts leading to feelings, feelings driving our actions, and actions determining our results. The thought cycle is an interconnected cycle that governs the outcomes we create in both business and life. When we work with our clients to guide them through their own thought cycles, they come to realize the core of how their minds work.

The value of connecting thoughts, emotions, and behaviors gives unparalleled insight into our mental framework. More than introspection, this work gives our clients a comprehensive map of their mental processes. Clients gain awareness of areas of potential roadblocks and detours that directly impact their level of success.

But the power of transformation is also revealed in that once clients spot these trends, they can then begin the work of shifting negative thoughts and beliefs into personal growth. This work molds and fashions an entrepreneurial mindset that is primed for success.

By mastering the power of our own thoughts, we are suited to craft the outcomes we desire most through purposeful and informed action that arises from an in-depth understanding of how our mentality directly impacts our achievements.

In essence, the thought cycle is an individual roadmap to success, guiding the individual to steer their business endeavors with clarity, focus, and a renewed sense of purpose.

Tool 4: Emotional Mastery: The Silent Force Behind Every Business Decision

Emotional mastery refers to the ability to understand, manage, and channel your emotions productively. It is not just about controlling emotions but the skillful direction or channeling of feelings to foster motivation, productivity, and success.

You've felt it. The surge of emotion that comes almost immediately after a lost deal or the euphoria of a breakthrough or major win. These emotions arise seemingly automatically after a particular outcome that may be desired or unwanted.

But imagine what is available to you when you create emotions ahead of time. The outcome that you wanted would be a natural progression of a process. Mastering emotions is not about suppression but channeling. Channeling is power. When you know how to create the emotions that fuel success, nothing is impossible to you. Being emotionally masterful is crucial for anyone looking to achieve their goals, especially entrepreneurs aiming for success in their ventures.

But before our clients can channel their emotions, they first need to understand them. We take them through a process of recognizing what they feel and why they feel it as the first step.

And the next step is learning to harness emotions to utilize them as fuel for ambition and productivity.

Once harnessed, emotions are then directed toward achieving business goals, fostering an environment of growth and achievement, and ultimately creating a life of purpose and fulfillment.

Self-care is pivotal to emotional understanding. It helps ground individuals, provides clarity, and reduces reactionary behaviors. Self-care encourages that rather than being overwhelmed by emotions, you can intentionally tap into them and channel feelings into constructive actions.

A fulfilling life and successful business await the entrepreneur who is able to align their emotional compass with their vision and allow their emotions to connect their passion with their purpose.

Thus, by mastering emotions, individuals unlock a potent tool that turns challenges into opportunities and ambitions into realities. Emotional mastery goes beyond introspection and self-awareness. It becomes a tangible strategy for success, where inner feelings are translated into measurable outcomes.

Emotions are powerful drivers of action. When harnessed correctly, they can propel individuals toward their dreams.

ACTIVITY

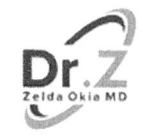

LIFE WHEEL
On a scale of 1-10 (10 being the highest)

Dr. Z
Zelda Okia MD

AREA OF LIFE	PRIORITY IN YOUR LIFE	LEVEL OF SATISFACTION	WHAT WOULD MAKE IT A 10?
RELATIONSHIPS			
EMOTIONAL HEALTH			
MONEY			
TIME			
PHYSICAL HEALTH			
CAREER			
SPIRITUAL PRACTICE			

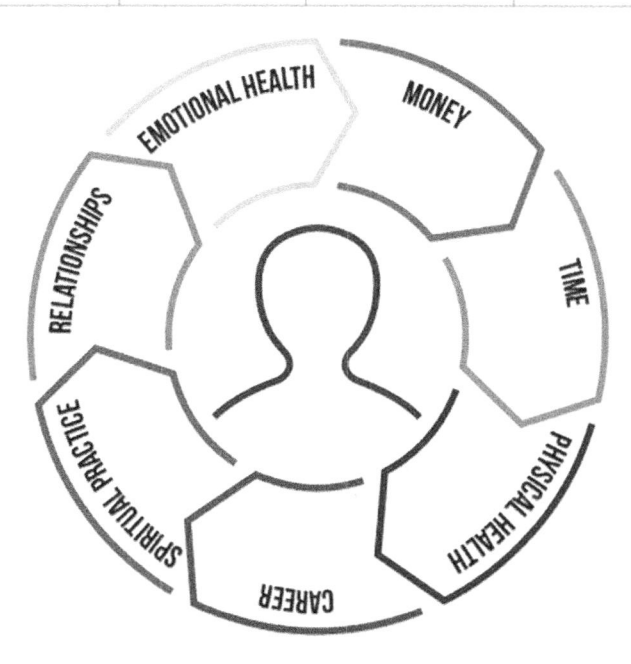

About the Author

Dr. Zelda Okia, or Dr. Z, presents a remarkable journey from an overwhelmed, overweight physician to a transformative life coach.

Several years ago, Dr. Z was a typical healthcare professional—dedicated to caring for others but struggling with personal health and wellness. Initially thin, her life changed after her medical training. Despite earning well, traveling, and dining at fine restaurants, she became increasingly unhappy and noticed significant weight gain. This realization led her to join a running club and undertake a 12-week weight loss program. However, her initial success was short-lived as she regained the weight, prompting her to seek a more sustainable solution. This quest led her to life coaching, where she found remarkable success. Under the guidance of her mentor coach, Dr. Z lost 30 pounds, a transformation she has maintained. This personal success inspired her to become a life coach, aiming to help others find peace and freedom around food.

Today, Dr. Z is dedicated to helping her clients transition from feeling overwhelmed and underappreciated to leading balanced, healthy lifestyles. She emphasizes sustainable weight loss, mental energy, and fitness through transformative self-care, believing firmly that one cannot give from an empty cup. Her expertise is further enriched by her part-time work as a forensic pathologist/medical examiner. This role has given her an intimate understanding of the detrimental effects of poor diet and unhealthy lifestyle choices.

Dr. Z's coaching approach focuses on developing consistent habits and self-mastery, enabling her clients to achieve significant life transformations. They not only lose weight and maintain it but also gain energy, vitality, and an overall abundant life. One of her notable successes involves a minister who found renewed joy in her vocation after participating in her program. This transformation occurred as the minister learned to detach from the burden of being responsible for others' spiritual experiences.

Dr. Z extends an invitation to join her transformative journey, promising physical well-being, mental clarity, healthy weight maintenance, and a fulfilling work-life balance. This journey is specially tailored for busy healthcare professionals, offering a path towards a more balanced and fulfilling life.

Email: zeldaokia@gmail.com
Website: www.zeldaokia.com
Facebook: https://www.facebook.com/zelda.okia
Instagram: @zeldaokia https://www.instagram.com/zeldaokia/
LinkedIN: https://www.linkedin.com/in/zelda-okia-md-b7a921184/
YouTube: https://www.youtube.com/@EasyWeightLoss411
Tik Tok: https://www.tiktok.com/@zeldaokia

CHAPTER 12

An Inside-Out Approach to Work-Life Balance

By Rebecca Olson
Life Coach for Working Moms, Podcast Host
Benicia, California

Balance isn't something you find, it's something you create.
—Jana Kingsford

As a coach for ambitious working moms, I teach that work-life balance is possible all of the time, in any job and in any life circumstance. Your clients don't need a different job, fewer responsibilities, a spouse that is more helpful, or a boss who is less demanding. Work-life balance is something your clients have the ability to control.

The reason I approach work-life balance in this way is that it's the most *useful* belief to have. If your client is thinking, "Work-life balance isn't possible in this job," their only option is to quit, even if they don't *want* to. When they believe that they control their work-life balance, it opens their mind up to solutions.

I had a client who was an accountant. When we first started working together, she told me tax season was always a time when she worked crazy hours and it felt like work-life balance was unattainable. If she continued to believe that work-life balance was found in the job or the season of the year, her only option would have been to slog through it and work obsessively through that season until it was over. But no one wants a life where balance is only possible half the year.

In this chapter, I will walk you through the four steps to attain a work-life balance that feels completely in your client's control. I formed this process after six years of coaching and teaching working moms what can often feel like an elusive and mysterious feeling of balance. In this chapter, I will take the mystery out of work-life balance.

What Is Balance?

I recently asked a group of working moms, "What is balance?" I received the typical response: a reasonable split of time between work, family, and self. While this answer is not entirely wrong, they were missing a key component of balance.

Think about how the word "balance" is often used: "I want to *feel* balanced." It is often thought of like it is a *feeling*, an emotional state. This means balance is not going to be found in a perfect set of circumstances; it will be found where all emotions are found: in the body.

This is an important point to understand, because if balance continues to be found in a perfect schedule, a helpful partner, the right number of friends, a manageable to-do list, a certain amount of money in savings, etc., then your client will burn out trying to get every piece of life in perfect order. I have clients who come to me working 60 hours a week, some that work 40 hours, and some are between jobs. All of them say they feel out of balance. The only way that is possible is if balance is found in something other than circumstance.

When you approach balance as an emotional state, how you help your clients changes dramatically. Cognitive behavioral theory indicates that there is a direct correlation between what you think and what you feel, which means if you want to *feel* balanced, then the solution is found, not in changing the circumstances but in changing the way you think.

Now, just changing your client's mindset is not going to be the complete process to create a life that feels balanced. In order to create a different life, they must *do* something different in addition to thinking differently. Your clients will need to learn skills in how to not always be available, say no, stop work at the time they want, schedule uninterrupted time for themselves, and not to schedule over personal priorities. But in order for someone to experience balance, these behavior changes will start with a shift in their mind.

Moving From a State of Imbalance to Balance

There are four steps to creating sustainable work-life balance: confidence, clarity, controlling the mind, and boundaries. To be the most effective, the steps should be followed in this order as they begin internally and extend externally.

Step 1: Confidence

My client, Katie, worked for a billionaire. This billionaire did amazing things for the planet. My client was really connected to the work she was doing, made a lot of money, adored her three amazing kids, and absolutely loved her marriage. Yet when we started coaching together, she told me, "I'm not happy. I feel like I should be happy. I have everything I want, but I'm not happy." The reason she wasn't experiencing the happiness that was possible for her was not about her life circumstances; it was what she was thinking about herself and those circumstances. She had endless negative chatter in her head, constantly telling her she wasn't enough, she wasn't doing enough, and she was letting people down. She felt guilty, lost, and inadequate.

The most important thoughts a client will need in order to feel balanced are the thoughts they have about themselves. Confidence is the belief in yourself. To create a life that feels balanced, your client must have a generally positive script running through their head about who they are.

Your client could be the best at their job, could get a raise every year, and could get consistently promoted. They could be named number one on their team and highly praised by everyone in the company. If *they* don't think they're great at what they do, they won't be confident. It's the way *they* think about themselves that is either going to make them feel amazing and successful, or not.

As you coach your clients on work-life balance, the first step will be to coach your clients on the thoughts they have about themselves and their lives. You want them to know and love themselves on the deepest level possible. This critical first step will allow them to make the eventual priority shifts necessary to make decisions about what is most important to them and then to protect those priorities even when it is hard.

Step 2: Clarity

The human brain craves direction. With only 24 hours in a day, your client will need to choose, with intentionality and purpose, how to spend that time. As the coach, you will help your client create a roadmap for their brain to know the direction to move. This is achieved by getting clear on what they want and why in the areas of their career and their priorities.

Clarity on Career Direction

Your client spends more hours working than any other activity in life. In order to feel balanced their brain needs to feel clear that the time spent working is worth it. Here's why: When work gets busy, it is hard to hold to boundaries. The most natural place for the brain to go is, "I can't do this, I should just quit, I need to find something new." This is a very common problem for the brain because it has an "all-in or all-out" approach to problems. The problem is, when their brain is thinking that the only way to create balance is to quit or to go part-time, what the brain is *not* doing is finding solutions for how to stay in the job and make more balanced choices.

My client, Ali, came to coaching after changing jobs four times. She kept thinking the next job would make her happy and allow her to experience the balance she wanted in life. Yet within four to six months, she would find herself overwhelmed and ready to find the next job. She thought the issue was the job, and she kept searching for the "right" one. The problem was, she didn't have a picture of the "right" job. She lacked clarity on what she wanted in a job and how her job fit into the bigger picture of the life she wanted to create. In coaching, we spent time getting clear on her career direction and priorities. We established her deeper values and strengths and thought long term about how she wanted her career to impact her life with her family. She was able to make some big decisions to move her family across the country and to go after a promotion in a different industry more aligned with where she wanted to take her career. She's still in that job today and feels happier and balanced.

Clarity on Daily Priorities

When your client arrives home from work, at least ten things are competing for their attention. If your client is not clear on which one of these tasks is the most important, they will default to the one that feels the most urgent but likely is not the most important.

When you help your clients decide ahead of time what their priorities are, they will start to make faster decisions that feel in alignment with what they want to achieve. I had a client who was a veterinarian. She was always stressed about two competing priorities: Get to as many patients as possible, or give quality care to her patients and to her patients' caregivers. We spent time in a session discussing each of these priorities and which one was the most important to her and why. In the end, she decided quality care was much more important than being on time. Although it didn't feel good to keep people waiting, she knew she was choosing the priority most important to her. Deciding that helped her feel centered and in control, even when it didn't always feel good.

Step 3: Controlling Your Mind

Your client's boss emails and says, "I need that report by tomorrow." They panic. "Oh no! I didn't know they needed that. I'm totally behind. I don't want to let them down!" So they stay late working on it, sacrificing their evening plans. Your client also could have thought, "Huh, I wonder if this could get pushed back?" This would leave them feeling curious, leading them to ask if the deadline could get moved. Or they could think, "Since

I don't want to work late tonight, what is the best way to tackle this, so I get the most done?" This would allow them to feel empowered and shut down all distractions, so they can be as productive as possible.

It is the client's perspective, or thoughts, that drive their decision to either work late, push back on the deadline, or problem-solve for how to get the work done. It is their thoughts that drive their decisions.

Remember there is a direct correlation between what you think, feel, and do. In order for your client to change imbalanced behaviors such as working late, checking messages, staying available after hours, and mindlessly scrolling social media, you will need to help your client understand the connection between how their thoughts drive these behaviors, so they can cultivate new ones.

My client, Jessica, had the hardest time leaving work on time. She desperately wanted to be home with her family for dinner and bedtime, but her brain kept telling her, "You didn't get enough done today. You should have done more. People are going to be disappointed in you." These thoughts left her feeling guilty and inadequate, so she worked late in order to get a little more done. But her tasks were endless and she never felt like she was doing a good job on top of feeling like she was failing her family by not being home on time. She was in a constant state of imbalance, feeling lost and stuck.

In coaching, I helped Jessica uncover her "not enough" thoughts and showed her how it was driving her actions. Together, we examined if she truly believed she wasn't doing enough and offered her brain new perspectives on how she was doing quite well in her role. She quickly started feeling more confident, and her "not enough" thoughts showed up less and less, allowing her to leave work on time with more ease.

In order for your clients to correct their overworking behavior, they will need to cultivate thoughts that make them feel calm and in control, so they take action from that new emotional state.

Step 4: Boundaries

Now that your client feels confident in who they are and are clear on their priorities, it's time to protect those priorities. Protecting priorities is most commonly called a boundary. This step is about learning to protect the things most important to your clients, regardless if someone is disappointed, not on board, or looks down on them for doing it, which is the hard part.

I teach my clients the only thing that gets in the way of them making a decision to uphold their boundary is an uncomfortable emotion. Guilt, disappointment, inadequacy, and fear of failure—these are at the heart of why your clients say yes to things that go against their priorities.

Jasmine had a boss who consistently asked for things on Friday afternoons. Before our coaching work, she would work over the weekend to deliver on the task because she didn't want him to be disappointed or think she wasn't a team player. This took away time from her family and left her exhausted because she wasn't honoring her rest time. Through coaching, she learned how to recognize the uncomfortable emotions that came up when upholding her boundaries, process them, and let them go. She stopped labeling her negative emotions as "bad" or "wrong," and she accepted that saying no doesn't always feel good, but that's okay.

As the coach, it is your job to help your clients stop avoiding their negative emotions and instead learn to feel them and let them go. Feelings are meant to be felt, not avoided, carried around as a heavy burden, or stuffed deep down and not seen. When someone mistreats their uncomfortable emotions, it leads to emotional exhaustion, explosions over little things, and a lack of control.

An important tool I use in my coaching practice that helps my clients process their emotions is a step-by-step guide on how to handle boundary-compromising moments that hold uncomfortable emotions. My suggested Boundary Protocol is at the end of this chapter and will act as a guide.

To conclude, sustainable work-life balance for a client is not about doing everything; it's about being selective with commitments and letting go of the rest. In order to achieve this, your client needs an unshakable view of themselves (confidence), an understanding of what is most important to them (clarity), and to honor those priorities, no matter how it feels (controlling the mind and boundaries). This inside-out approach has your client focused on what they can control: themselves.

ACTIVITY

Boundary Protocol

This protocol is meant to be followed when you have made a commitment that you find yourself compromising on because it feels hard or uncomfortable, someone else may be disappointed, or you fear what others think. For example:

- Ending work at 5:30 p.m.
- Not logging on after the kids have gone to sleep
- Holding to your "heads down" time and not moving the meeting around
- Leaving emails and messages unread during "heads down" time

This is exactly what I want you to do in the moment when you find yourself deciding if you are going to follow through and hold to your commitment/boundary and a wave of emotion overcomes you.

In the past, this wave of emotion would normally derail you and have you compromising on what you'd planned to do, but following this protocol will help you follow through.

1. **STOP**: Stop what you are doing.
2. **NOTICE**: Notice the feeling that has just flooded your body (fear, inadequacy, uncertainty, insecurity, etc.).
3. **NORMALIZE**: Say out loud, "I see [feeling] has entered my body. Yes, it makes sense that this would show up right now. It's okay."
4. **BREATHE**: Take deep breaths in and out until you notice the sensations start to "soften" or dissipate (30 seconds to 2 minutes).

5. **INTENTIONAL THINKING**: Remind your brain why you have this boundary/commitment and why you are sticking to it by answering one of these questions (or come up with your own):

- *How do I know this is the right thing to do?*
- *Why do I want to stick to this commitment?*
- *What do I gain from sticking to this commitment?*
- *What does my family gain?*
- *How am I certain things will be okay?*
- *How do I know I am safe and secure?*
- *What am I in control of right now?*

6. **ACTION**: Follow through with the commitment/boundary IN THE MOMENT while your brain is calm and on board. Don't delay it.

About the Author

Rebecca Olson is an international life coach, speaker, and podcast host who helps career-focused parents stop feeling overwhelmed and "not enough" so they can be present with their kids while crushing their career goals.

Through her coaching programs and top-ranking podcast, *Ambitious and Balanced Working Moms*, Rebecca has helped tens of thousands of parents learn to feel confident in who they are, what they want, and the value they bring to their company and family. She teaches an inside-out approach to creating a work-life balance that gives individuals control over their time, energy, and success.

Rebecca is known for her straight talk and big earrings. She lives in the San Francisco Bay Area with her husband and two kiddos. When not coaching or speaking, she loves playing ultimate frisbee and drinks lots of tea.

Website: www.rebeccaolsoncoaching.com
LinkedIn: https://www.linkedin.com/in/rebolson/
Instagram: https://www.instagram.com/rebeccaolsoncoach/

CHAPTER 13

Navigating Early Adult Life Transitions

By Anna Pagliuca, MSc
Life and Mental Health Coach
Utrecht, Netherlands

The panic years. That's how my twenties have felt anyway. A panic to be perfect, to have everything figured out before 30 ... Quite frankly, I'm tired of panicking over the panic years, but I know I'm gonna continue to panic over them anyway.

—Elle Louise Wilmont

Life is a series of transitions. From the moment we take our first breath to the last, our existence unfolds through a continuous series of changes. Some are gradual and imperceptible, like the ever-turning seasons, while others are sudden and transformative, like a bolt of lightning in a darkened sky. Early adulthood, that nebulous phase between the exuberance of youth and the responsibilities of maturity, is a period when the echoes of childhood dreams meet the realities of grown-up choices, shaping the course of one's life in ways both exhilarating and daunting.

The transitions that characterize early adulthood hold a significance that cannot be overstated. They are the milestones of self-discovery, identity formation, and the forging of one's path in the world. Early adult life transitions encompass a diverse array of experiences—from leaving the nest and starting college or a career, to forming meaningful relationships and grappling with existential questions.

Each transition brings its unique set of challenges, joys, and revelations. It is a time when young adults step out of their comfort zones, leave their familiar homes, and embark on a journey toward independence. It is a time filled with dreams and aspirations. The anticipation of newfound freedom, making new friends, and exploring uncharted territories can be exhilarating. However, alongside this excitement, there's often an undercurrent of uncertainty—adapting to a new routine, managing finances, coping with academic or work pressures, dealing with the feeling of being alone in a sea of strangers.

In this chapter, we will delve into the multifaceted nature of early adult life transitions, and what we, as coaches, can do to help individuals coming to us with these issues.

The transition to college life or work life can indeed be an emotional rollercoaster, marked by a range of highs and lows. In both my personal life and working with young adults, I have noticed there are specific emotional stages that often accompany these early adult life transitions. First, as the transition period approaches, there's a palpable sense of anticipation and excitement. Whether it's heading off to college or starting a new job, the prospect of new experiences, independence, and the unknown future can be exhilarating. Dreams and aspirations abound, and optimism runs high. Alongside excitement, anxiety and apprehension often rear their heads. The unknown can be daunting, and leaving behind the familiar—be it home, friends, or routines—can trigger anxiety. Questions about fitting in, meeting expectations, and handling newfound responsibilities can keep one up at night.

Once the transition begins, there's a period of adjustment and adaptation. In college, this may involve navigating a new campus, managing coursework, and making friends. In the workplace, it might entail learning new job tasks and adapting to the professional environment. This phase can be marked by moments of both triumph and frustration as individuals find their footing. For many, transitioning to college or work means being away from the support system they've relied on for years. Feelings of homesickness and loneliness can be profound during this time. The longing for the familiarity of home, family, and friends can be emotionally challenging. With time and experience, confidence begins to build. In college, students gain a sense of autonomy in managing their studies and daily lives. In the workplace, new employees start to take ownership of their roles and responsibilities. This newfound independence can be empowering and boost self-esteem.

As responsibilities mount and the novelty of the transition wears off, stress and pressure may increase. College students juggle coursework, exams, and extracurricular activities, while young professionals face deadlines, expectations, and workplace dynamics. The pressure to perform and succeed can lead to stress-related emotions.

Amidst the challenges, there is also a period of exploration and self-discovery. College students explore new subjects, hobbies, and relationships. Young professionals discover their strengths and weaknesses, passions, and career goals. These moments of self-discovery can be deeply fulfilling and exciting. Over time, individuals often develop resilience and grow stronger. They learn to adapt to setbacks, manage stress more effectively, and build support networks. The rollercoaster of emotions begins to level out as they become more accustomed to their new life circumstances. Finally, as individuals settle into their college or work life, they often experience a sense of fulfillment and satisfaction. Achieving academic or career milestones, forming meaningful relationships, and pursuing personal goals can bring a deep sense of contentment.

A coach can be incredibly valuable for someone who is transitioning into adulthood. We saw how this period of life is often filled with significant changes and challenges, and a life coach can provide guidance, support, and tools to help individuals navigate this transition successfully. There are various important tasks coaches can assist with and guide in. By offering personalized guidance and support, a life coach empowers individuals to face the challenges of this phase and thrive in various aspects of their lives.

One of the key roles of a life coach is helping individuals define their goals, encompassing academic, career, personal development, and relationship aspirations. This process involves not only setting these goals but also creating a strategic plan to achieve them, which might include education choices, job search skills, and interview preparation. Boosting self-confidence and self-esteem is another vital aspect of a life coach's role. By instilling a positive mindset, individuals can approach challenges with resilience and determination.

Life coaches also focus on imparting essential life skills, including time management, financial literacy, communication, and problem-solving abilities. These skills are fundamental for navigating the complexities of adulthood successfully. Managing stress and anxiety is a common struggle during this transition. A life coach equips individuals with coping mechanisms and stress-reduction techniques, enabling them to effectively handle the pressures of life.

Additionally, life coaches assist in developing and maintaining healthy relationships, both personally and professionally, by honing communication skills, conflict resolution abilities, and boundary-setting techniques. Financial literacy is emphasized to ensure individuals understand budgeting, saving, investing, and managing debt, promoting financial independence and stability.

Moreover, life coaches guide individuals in establishing holistic lifestyle habits, encompassing diet, exercise, sleep, and mental well-being. Decision-making skills are honed through coaching, enabling individuals to make informed and confident choices about education, career, relationships, and other life aspects. Life coaches also serve as accountability partners, helping individuals stay focused on their goals by providing motivation and encouragement. Navigating significant life transitions, such as moving to a new city, changing careers, or starting a family, can be challenging. Life coaches provide practical strategies and emotional support to ease these transitions.   Furthermore, fostering self-reflection is a core component of coaching. Life coaches facilitate this process, helping individuals gain insights into their strengths, values, and passions, which are invaluable for personal growth. Inevitably, failures and setbacks are part of adulthood. Life coaches teach resilience skills, enabling individuals to bounce back from these challenges, emerge stronger, and continue their journey toward personal and professional fulfillment. Through personalized guidance and tailored support, life coaches empower individuals to make confident decisions, overcome obstacles, and thrive during the transition into adulthood. This personalized approach ensures that coaching sessions are highly effective and impactful in addressing the unique needs and challenges of each individual.

In the world of coaching, there's a handy tool called the "coach matrix." The coach matrix is part of what we refer to as strategic coaching, a personalized and goal-oriented approach that focuses on helping individuals achieve specific objectives, resulting in an actionable plan for the coachee to implement after the coaching journey. In strategic coaching, a coach works closely with the client to define clear, achievable goals and develop a structured plan to reach those goals. Unlike general coaching, which may cover a wide range of topics, strategic coaching is highly focused and tailored to address specific challenges or goals. Therefore, strategic coaching centers around specific, targeted questions related to decision-making. Strategic coaching can be applied in various contexts, such as personal development, career advancement, leadership skills enhancement, and organizational performance improvement. In this case, individuals who are undergoing early adult life transitions may seek guidance on managing stress, contemplating a career/study change, considering relocation, or creating new friendships and connections.

In this type of coaching, the coach matrix acts like a map guiding you through the maze of thoughts and emotions. Imagine it as a clear path, helping you understand yourself and others better. This matrix is a structured approach that lends clarity to the often-complex world of human thoughts and emotions. It structures the guidance process, infusing it with a sense of order and purpose. By following its systematic path, you empower your clients to shape their own destinies, fostering autonomy in their personal evolution. Together, you dissect the core questions:

1. What are the facts?
2. What is your problem or question?
3. What is your goal?
4. What action will you take?

Each of the four questions is meant to serve a specific purpose:

- Challenging assumptions: What are the fundamental truths underlying your beliefs?

- Defining the question: What issue or query is at the core, whether personal, relational, or systemic?
- Envisioning the goal: What does success look like, often standing in stark contrast to the problem at hand?
- Planning action: What steps will you take to bridge the gap between your current state and your envisioned success?

Ultimately, the coach matrix embedded in the strategic coaching approach is aimed at empowering individuals to make strategic decisions, maximize their potential, and achieve meaningful and sustainable results.

As we conclude this chapter, remember this: The knowledge you've gained here isn't just information; it's a catalyst for transformation. Armed with the coach matrix, you possess new tools to guide yourself and others toward autonomy and self-realization. You have the ability to inspire change, foster growth, and nurture resilience. In the realm of coaching and guidance, these tools aren't just assets; they are beacons of hope. They illuminate the way forward, not just for your clients, but for you as well. As you apply these principles, you become not just a coach or a guide, but a facilitator of transformation.

ACTIVITY

See the Coach Matrix within the chapter.

About the Author

Anna Pagliuca, a professional hailing from Italy, is a versatile individual with a passion for psychology and mental health. Having lived in Italy, the USA, and the Netherlands, she possesses a global perspective that enriches her understanding of diverse cultures and lifestyles. Anna holds a bachelor's degree in psychology and a master's degree in clinical psychology, reflecting her dedication to the field.

Since March 2023, Anna has been making a meaningful impact as a mental health coach, specializing in guiding young adults toward better mental well-being. Her empathetic approach and extensive knowledge empower her clients to navigate the challenges of early adulthood successfully.

Driven by her commitment to helping others, Anna is currently undergoing advanced training to become a psychotherapist, aiming to deepen her expertise and broaden her capacity to support individuals facing mental health issues. With her unique blend of academic prowess and real-world experience, Anna is dedicated to making a positive difference in the lives of those she encounters.

Email: annarosariapagliuca@gmail.com
LinkedIn: https://www.linkedin.com/in/anna-pagliuca-13ba81200/

CHAPTER 14

Transforming Stress into Strength: Insights and Strategies for Coaches

By David Pasikov
Executive, Business, and Life Coach, Psychotherapist
Big Rapids, Michigan

*The greatest weapon against stress is our ability
to choose one thought over another.*

—William James

Stress As a Way of Life

For many clients who seek out coaching, stress can be a way of life. From the personal or professional stressors they face routinely, to the real or perceived challenges and obstacles in their lives, coaching clients (think of coaching as an adjective) require solid skills and strategies to help manage and alleviate stress. Clearly, then, it's essential that we as coaches are adept at addressing our clients' stress, whenever and however it appears.

Most of us are well-versed in the fight, flight, or freeze responses people have when experiencing stress. Several years ago, I was in a session with a man who grew up in New York City, surrounded by rival gangs and no stranger to violence. During our session, the sun began to shine in my eyes from the window behind him and, without announcing my intent, I got out of my chair and walked beside him to lower the blind. As I approached him, I noticed that my client moved his body away from me and made his hand into a fist. I quietly sat down and asked him if he'd noticed what had just occurred. His response was so automatic that he had no idea he'd reacted that way. That gave us a handle into his survival mechanism and threat response. Asking clients about both their stress levels and their stress management techniques can be central to the coaching process. This is valuable information as it can seem next to impossible to make lasting changes when unmanaged stress is blocking a client's path.

Because we are going to encounter clients who are stressed and even traumatized, let's take a moment to look at the difference between the two. With stress, its symptoms generally diminish when a threat (whether real or perceived) is eliminated. With trauma, however, symptoms can linger indefinitely, long after a traumatic event has passed. It is important to be able to make this distinction, as unpacking trauma can require a very specific set of therapeutic skills. Even seasoned psychotherapists often will choose to refer clients to a trauma specialist, and, as coaches, we are wise to err on the side of making such a referral. Often, too, clients can continue with the coaching process while separately addressing their trauma with a qualified therapist.

The Biology of Stress

Before we explore how to resource our clients in managing their stress, let's take a deeper dive into the biology of stress.

Imagine yourself speeding to work on a busy highway. Suddenly, a reckless driver cuts in front of you, nearly causing a collision, and gives you a rude gesture out their window. Even though you are a sophisticated member of the 21st century, the same primal mechanism that kept your distant ancestors alive kicks in for you. You have a biological response to the perceived threat, except that you are hurtling down the highway, and you can't safely freeze. You can go into road rage and attempt to fight your perpetrator or engage in a flight response by getting off at the next exit, but most likely you are simply stuck in your car, stewing in your own chemicals.

Any perceived threat can trigger this mechanism. We can be at home and receive a message to call our tax preparer—and suddenly we are in fight, flight, or freeze, waiting for the bad news. When we call back and are informed that they have discovered a way to save us $500 on our taxes, we breathe a sigh of relief, and we have to recalibrate our autonomic nervous system from this false alarm. If we have a sustained period of real threats or even false alarms, our autonomic nervous system can keep firing—and we can be what is called "sympathetic nervous system dominant." In other words, our survival mechanism and its biochemicals can stay stuck in the "on" position, keeping us hypervigilant and poised to spring into action. This can lead to taxing our minds and bodies, and even to illness—but as you will read later in this chapter, it doesn't have to be that way.

Anything we can do to stay in our calm center will serve us well and will also help our clients to do the same. Because the pressures our clients often experience in their professional and/or personal lives sometimes can seem overwhelming, bringing our attention to their stress is a key element. Whether I am working with my own stress or helping another with theirs, for me the antidotes to fight, flight, or freeze are as follows:

- Replacing "fight" with approaching the challenge proactively and creatively, instead of wasting energy in blaming myself or others;
- Replacing "flight" with facing the facts, no matter how humbling they may be; and,
- Replacing "freeze" by exploring options and forming an action plan to meet the challenge.

Transforming Stress into Strength

In 1970, Alvin Toffler authored the book *Future Shock*, in which he foretold how the future would bring an accelerated rate of technological and social change. The most succinct definition of future shock is a personal perception of "too much change in too short a period of time." Toffler also coined the term "information overload." I doubt that anyone would argue that his predictions have come true. The challenge—and the opportunity—is to live our life facing these demands effectively.

To help us transform our 21st century stresses into strengths, we can draw on the workings of a 19th century heating system for insight. In the early 1980s, I lived in a 100-year-old farmhouse in rural New Hampshire. The property had a woodlot, which we logged to heat the house. The system used hot water that was heated by an antique wood-fired boiler. The hot water would then circulate through the pipes to heat old-fashioned radiators in rooms throughout the house.

On a chilly day, as we stoked the fire, pressure would build up inside the boiler. Because the thermostat in the house was calling for heat, a valve would open and hot water would circulate through the radiators, which heated the house while also relieving the pressure in the boiler.

On a mild day, if we put too much wood into the boiler, the house was not calling for heat so the valve was closed. To safeguard the boiler, another valve would open, and the room next to the furnace room would overheat to the point of feeling like a sauna.

In heating terms, this was called the "dump zone" as all that unusable heat was dumped there to prevent the boiler from exploding. This was a waste of energy as well as the labor that went into cutting and moving the wood, but it stopped the boiler from destroying the house and us with it. And if eventually the dump zone was insufficient to discharge the pressure in the boiler, a safety valve on top of the boiler would blow. This filled the furnace room with steam, and the boiler would literally sound like a two-ton tea kettle.

One day while I was putting wood on the fire, I realized that this was a perfect analogy for stress management. Rather than heat as the pressure source, our clients have myriad sources of stress, such as unfulfilling work, the challenges of child-rearing, financial pressures . . . the list can go on and on. Regardless of the stressors, when pressure builds up, it can cause an overload. Coaching our clients on how to creatively channel these pressures can be an invaluable tool in navigating life.

The following diagram illustrates how this model can work in a hypothetical coaching situation:

Example of How to Use the Boiler as a Stress Management Tool

E) Safety Valve: Spouse, Friend, Exercise, Reading, Music, Bath, Mindfulness, Self-Care

C) Creative Channel for Release:	B) Pressure (Energy) Anger Frustration Despair	D) Dump Zone	Dumping on Others = A) Accusation B) Blame C) Criticism
Meet with Manager		Dump on Others: That's not my job. Ask Bob!!! You're to blame for all of our money issues!!!	Dump on Self: I can't do anything right. I have no willpower.	NOTE: These are the ABCs of Ineffective Communication
Talk with spouse & set up a budget				
Change my diet & start exercising				Dumping on Self = A) Self-Accusation B) Self-Blame C) Self-Criticism

A) Heat Source (Source of Stress):

| Demanding Manager |
| Increased Medical Bills |
| Health Challenges |

To transform stress into strength, we need to:
A) Identify the sources of stress
B) Understand the pressures that the stress brings
C) Harness the pressure creatively
D) Avoid wasting the energy by dumping on others or self
E) Use our safety valves to nurture ourselves and help regulate the pressures.

© 2023 David Pasikov

Let's walk through the above example.

A. Rather than wood as the heat source, now we have various sources of stress, such as a demanding manager, financial pressures, etc.
B. This builds up pressure in us, which can be seen as energy, such as anger, despair, etc.
C. We can channel that energy creatively by meeting with our manager, talking with our spouse, etc.
D. For me, the ABCs of ineffective communication are accusation, blame, and criticism. I have listed examples in the sections entitled, "Dump on Others" and "Dump on Self."
E. The safety valve section has some examples of activities that can be done to take the pressure off creatively, which will differ from person to person. Note: In the boiler, the safety valve was the last resort, but in using this model personally, you can employ the safety valve at any time.

The bottom line is that when we are in the dump zone, we are in "victim" mode. We are at a standstill, and we are making matters worse by allowing unchecked pressure to continue to build. We've all seen clients at a standstill, and, of course, we all have intense feelings. What we do with them is where the power is. Self-empowerment in the face of stress *is*

Transforming Stress into Strength: Insights and Strategies for Coaches

achievable through creatively channeling our stressors and regulating life's pressures through our personal safety valves.

The following is a blank worksheet for you to use on your own or as a tool with your clients.

Boiler Diagram Worksheet

3   E) Safety Valve: _____ _____ _____ _____ _____ _____

C) Creative Channel for Release:

1 → B) Pressure (Energy) ∠ 2   D) Dump Zone

Dump on Others: Dump on Self:

A) Heat Source (Source of Stress):

Dumping on Others =
A) Accusation
B) Blame
C) Criticism

NOTE: These are the ABCs of Ineffective Communication

Dumping on Self =
A) Self-Accusation
B) Self-Blame
C) Self-Criticism

To transform stress into strength, we need to:
A) Identify the sources of stress
B) Understand the pressures that the stress brings
C) Harness the pressure creatively
D) Avoid wasting the energy by dumping on others or self
E) Use our safety valves to nurture ourselves and help regulate the pressures.

© 2023 David Pasikov

When a client needs help managing stress, putting it all together looks like this:

A) Identify the source(s) of stress.
B) Acknowledge and understand the pressures stress brings.
C) Harness the pressure creatively.
D) Avoid wasting energy by dumping on yourself or others.
E) Identify and use safety valves to help regulate life's pressures.

Stress Is Not the Enemy

Ask a room full of people to raise their hands if they believe stress can make them sick, and nearly every hand will go up. Then ask if stress can kill them, and watch how many hands remain in the air. Dr. Joe Dispenza, whose groundbreaking research on the mind/body relationship has resulted in fascinating recommendations regarding meditation and wellness writes, "Every time we make a thought, we make a chemical. If we have good thoughts, we have chemicals that make us feel good. And if we have negative thoughts, we have chemicals that make us feel exactly the way that we are thinking." So how do we help our clients change the way they think as they navigate the path to changing their lives for the better?

It is worthy of note that Hans Selye, widely regarded as the father of stress research, delineated two categories of stress: *distress* which negatively affects us, and *eustress* which has a positive effect on us. While distress unchecked can lead to disease and despair, eustress supports our physical health, mental performance, and emotional well-being.

The way I explain it to my clients is that we each have an internal two-drawer pharmacy cabinet. The lower drawer is labeled "Distress Chemicals." If we allow our perceptions and perspectives to open this drawer, we release stress hormones such as adrenaline, cortisol, and norepinephrine, which in the short term can help us cope with a threat but in the long term can tax our system.

The top drawer of our internal pharmacy cabinet is labeled "Eustress Chemicals." When we open this drawer, we release the healing hormones of dopamine, serotonin, oxytocin, and endorphins, all of which play a role in how we experience happiness, health, and well-being. When we are a creative channel for release and acting as our own safety valve, we are releasing these healing chemicals. At any given moment, we each have a choice: either open the *distress* drawer or the *eustress* drawer. But how do we guide ourselves and our clients to consistently make the better choice?

Einstein once said, "The most important decision we make is whether we believe we live in a friendly or hostile universe." Based on my client's intrinsic response to my walking beside him unannounced, we all can guess what he believed about the world. And many of us have seen the vicious cycle such thinking can create, whether in ourselves or in others. When we release distress chemicals in response to life's stressors, we are changing the way our brain and body perceive and respond to stress. That response in turn releases more of those chemicals, and the cycle continues. So, what is the answer?

Emerging research tells us that the key to shifting from distress to eustress may lie in something accessible to us all: *Gratitude*. This came to focus in my life in 2019 when I fell from a step ladder while changing a furnace filter. I will spare you the details, but I seriously injured both legs and hit my head. As I was lying on the floor unable to move either leg, I took an inventory and found that I could still wiggle my toes, and I determined that I didn't have a head injury.

It was such a freak accident that I realized that there was a powerful message here. At that moment, I recalled a seven-word phrase that a very wise older man shared with me when I was in my 20s: "Thankful for all things under all circumstances." This phrase has powerfully served me over the years as I have grown to see that my greatest challenges invariably turn out to be my greatest opportunities for growth. That phrase coming to mind gave me pause to reflect on my situation. I have plenty of data to unequivocally show me that I live in a friendly universe, something for which I am perpetually grateful. This way of thinking shifted me to absolutely avoid the dump zone, which freed me at that moment to not go into "victim."

I've used the boiler model to navigate life's challenges since the '80s. The ladder crisis put that to the test like never before. I spent two months in a rehab hospital after surgery, bedridden and locked in leg braces to heal the quadriceps tendons in both legs, along with a broken ankle and a badly sprained one.

I decided to be my own best client and use all the tools I have to manage my stress and support my healing. When I walked out of the rehab hospital after a two-month stay, I was told by the staff they expected my recovery to take far longer than it did. Never underestimate the power of transforming stress into strength.

Gratitude was a powerful key to my healing because it allowed me to focus on the positives in my circumstances. As coaches, we have to start with where the person is and then identify where they want to be. Closing that gap is my job as a coach. Helping the person move from the dump zone of blaming themselves or others for their life circumstances is an important step toward self-empowerment. When the time is right, supporting the person in having gratitude and seeing the silver lining in their circumstances is an important aspect of the coaching process.

People get paid in accordance with the level of problems that they can solve. I do not begrudge my orthopedic surgeon any money that he was paid. Without his training and skill in repairing and reattaching my quadriceps tendons, I would have spent the rest of my life in a wheelchair, unable to stand or take a step. As coaches, we are paid to help our clients close the gap between where they are and where they want to be, and in the process we help them address what they need to do to move their lives forward. Facing those challenges can be very stressful for our clients, and as a result, transforming stress into strength is fundamental to what we do.

The New Science of Stress

Several years ago, I learned of fascinating new research into the impact of stress on our lives. It is research that has fundamentally changed my thinking about stress in my own life and has led me to address my clients' perceptions of stress in a different way as well. The concepts that emerged are best encapsulated in a lecture by health psychologist Kelly McGonigal, who in a riveting TedTalk explains how it is not stress *per se* that affects us so profoundly but rather our *beliefs* about stress that dictate its impact on our lives. I highly recommend this lecture to my clients. I will end, in fact, with McGonigal's own words, because I believe they may resonate deeply with the important work that you, as a coach, have chosen to do in the world:

> *I wouldn't necessarily ask for more stressful experiences in my life, but this science has given me a whole new appreciation for stress … One thing we know for certain is that chasing meaning is better for your health than trying to avoid discomfort. And so I would say that's really the best way to make decisions, go after what it is that creates meaning in your life, and then trust yourself to handle the stress that follows.*

ACTIVITY

See Boiler Diagram worksheet within chapter.

About the Author

David Pasikov began his career as a science teacher in urban Detroit. With that foundation, he helped found and later became the executive director of a residential school for troubled teens in Ontario, Canada. From there, David went into a 25-year-long private practice as a psychotherapist in Boulder, Colorado, which included serving a term as president of the Colorado Association of Psychotherapists.

From 2005 to 2018, David taught advanced communication courses to senior executives and managers in the international high-tech sector. One of those courses was entitled "Leaders as Coaches." David ultimately realized that coaching would be an ideal next step in his career path, and he went on to earn his certification as a coach. He has since worked with a wide spectrum of clients—from college students to couples in crisis, and from a former Heisman Trophy winner to a Silicon Valley innovation pioneer—in all aspects of life, relationship, and business coaching.

David and his wife, Susan, live in Big Rapids, Michigan, where he continues his coaching practice while also serving as the U.S. coordinator of Life Alignment, a system he uses to help clients remove blockages in their lives and reach their full potential. For more information, visit www.life-alignment.com.

Email: david@pasikov.com
Website: www.pasikov.com

CHAPTER 15

Cultivating Transformational Coaching: Harnessing the Power of Vision and Values

By Anna Prinz
Life Coach; Founder of *The Crossroads Coach*
High Wycombe, England, United Kingdom

When values, thoughts, feelings and actions are in alignment, a person becomes focused and character is strengthened.
—John C. Maxwell

Cultivating and Harnessing

"Cultivating" is a horticultural term. It means to prepare the land for crops. It involves knowing what you want to grow and how that crop grows best in what type of soil and under what circumstances. It takes time, patience, and skill. As a great coach, you will ask questions that "prepare the land."

Cultivation in terms of coaching will involve preparation of the inner soil. If we run towards results as a coach, before digging deeper, we will end up like the farmer standing at the side of the field without any fruit.

To cultivate transformation in your clients, you must invite them to work through the soil, consider the nutrients already present, think about what else they need, and decide what kind of crop they want. What takes root? What grows well? What type of fruit is produced?

In other words, a great coach prepares the client for great results by inviting them to consider their inner world. What strengths does the client have? What beliefs are held on to? What do they *really* want? What is important in the process?

Transformational coaching is about *becoming the person* who is able to achieve the desired outcome. It is not about focusing only on the goal. The question is not "How do you achieve the result?" but "How do you become the person who can do this?" External force and dangling carrots that push us to do things that we think we ought to do but keep putting off will never offer the lasting and life-changing results that internal growth and the intrinsic motivation of transformational coaching offer.

Transformation focused on our inner world will then determine what our outer world looks like. Transformational coaching brings deep and long-lasting results due to the exploration of the inner world of vision and values. This chapter will explore why vision and values are so key to building a great coaching experience.

"Harnessing" is an industrial term meaning "to control and make use of … especially to produce energy." In terms of coaching, a great coach will lead the client to gain control over their own choices by bringing attention to what they deeply want and deem important in life. A great coach seeks to raise the energy of their client so that motivation increases to follow through with action. A great coach harnesses the inner power of vision and values to move forward with greater clarity, focus, and momentum. This chapter looks at how you can do that.

Vision is what I can see or what I visualise in my mind's eye. It is what I focus on and what I direct myself towards. For example, if I have the vision to become a doctor, I will study sciences at school and apply to study medicine. My vision determines what I aim for and in which direction I go. It also determines what I don't choose to do and what I actively turn away from.

Values are what are important to me, what I give time to, and what I prioritise. When I become aware of what is important to me, it gives me agency over my choices. I no longer choose based on what I want to avoid due to fear, but I choose based on my life values. That is integrity. And that is transformational.

My values determine how I walk on my journey, what I take, and what I consider a meaningful path. For example, if I value connection, my journey will involve companions whose company I enjoy. If I value making memories, I might take a camera. If I value kindness, I may bring along gifts for my companions.

Vision

Vision guides the outcome of the journey. As a great coach, you will guide the client to understand *where* they are going, *why* they are going there, and *how* to get there. A great coach invites the client to understand what they *really* want (desires) and orientate them towards it (direction) by helping them to gain clarity on where they are going (destination).

Desires—What Do You Really Want?

The heart wants what it wants. A great coach asks questions so that the client can clearly see their own heart, and a great coach walks beside them in support while they learn to live from their heart. Any other choice is fear-based.

When it comes down to it, we either pursue joy or try to avoid pain. It is so important for the coach to drill down to the client's true desires because any other basis will result in people-pleasing, hiding, and living below potential. Having said that, even when desires are clearly understood, the gap between what we see in the distance and what we see in front of our eyes today can loom large. As long as we don't move towards the vision we see, we can maintain the fantasy of the vision and it remains a possibility. The desires remain in our head. But our desires to add meaning and contribute to the world niggle away at the internal vision.

A great coach invites attention on the horizon and not on the gap between the now and the not yet. A great coach will create the first step towards the vision, and the client's energy comes from walking in alignment with values towards the vision. A great coach will assist in bringing the vision to life, rather like a midwife. A great coach invites the client to get excited about the possibilities and the joy involved and the integrity of aligning with values instead of reacting to the fear of "I can't get there" and "I don't know if I have it in me to try." We have reasons to move forward, and we have reasons to stay put. This is how you harness the vision and bring it into reality—the desire for the vision must become stronger than the desire to remain safe. The vision may be compelling, but if people's approval is also a driver, then the vision may stay just out of reach while the client subconsciously works on remaining safe, which is a deep human need important to recognise. The vision must become more compelling than the fear of failure. As a great coach, you will gently probe whether the client is believing lies. As a great coach, you will raise awareness of the push and pull of the various desires. Small forward steps will reveal the benefits of the vision and create momentum.

The key to unlock the client's potential is to find out what they really want and why.

Direction—How Do You Get There?

Setting the direction means how we go about accomplishing the task of reaching the desired destination. It is crucial to establish how we move towards our target; otherwise, we simply don't move! Setting out on an unfamiliar road (however passionate we feel about the outcome) can be daunting. We want to be seen as competent and accomplished. We want to avoid other people's judgement. And that's why we procrastinate. But it makes no difference how loudly we jump up and down about our amazing vision if we don't start towards it. A great coach supports the client to take small, manageable steps to keep moving forward. Motivation follows action and not the other way around. So, a great coach will keep the client moving with action steps that are aligned with their values.

Self-esteem is boosted when we keep commitments to ourselves. And motivation is generated when progress is made. In setting the direction, it is important to note that feeling motivated is not enough to move. Taking action is what produces results. So, get the client to focus on small actions that chip away at the wall, and they will look back to see how much has been achieved.

Within the direction set, do we see opportunities or obstacles? The answer will depend on how effectively we overcome our fear. A great coach will keep the client focused on the benefits of the vision, turning potential obstacles into learning points and opportunities into action plans.

The key is to keep moving forwards in the same direction.

Destination—Know Where You Are Going

Our vision speaks to us of where we want to go. Desire shows us why. Direction tells us how. And destination shows us where. The destination is the desired outcome of our steps in that direction. Imagine stopping to ask for directions on a path and asking, "Am I going in the right direction?" It makes no sense unless we can determine what our endpoint is. A great coach works with the client to firm up their goal. A great coach has a client who can say, "Yes, I am going in the right direction because I know where I am going."

How does a great coach harness the power of the destination? Keep it current. A client who lives it, breathes it, and sees their destination in their mind's eye regularly will daily be taking steps on the road to that destination. It matters not if the steps are small. Or even if the steps sometimes pause. What matters is that the client takes steps on the road to their desired place. Vision boards, sticky notes, voice messages, photos, book covers—creative ways to keep the vision tangible and within reach.

The key is to know what your destination is.

Values

Values guide how we live. As a great coach you will guide the client to understand *what* they consider important, *why* it is important, and *how* that makes the difference to all their decisions and habits. As a great coach, you will invite your client to understand how they get going (inspiration), what the priorities are (important), and what difference it is making (impact).

Inspiration—How Are You Motivated?

Before setting off towards the vision, a great coach invites the client to consider how best to start the journey. It's vital to know what gives us energy. This energy will compel us forwards towards our goal. Positive motivation moves us towards progress, benefits, achievement, success, self-esteem, contribution, making a difference, celebration, and joy. A great coach asks questions to elicit how the client interprets all of these and what they will actively do to reach towards them.

We are also motivated to avoid failure, pain, frustration, confusion, and incompetence. Motivated by these, the client stagnates. Negative motivation keeps people safe, but it keeps them trapped in the procrastination cycle. A great coach will bring awareness of this tendency but will focus on the positive to elicit momentum in the client.

How do you harness the inspiration? Focus on questions that will raise understanding of the benefits, define success and achievement, and explore what contribution and nuggets of joy along the way look like. The client gains energy from understanding the purpose of the goal. Fuel to provide that energy also comes from evidence-based strengths. A great coach invites the client to consider their previous strengths and to bring them to the current reality.

Fuel converting into energy still comes to nothing without the correct harnessing. Unless the client channels their inspiration, they are like a balloon whizzing around the room, expelling air but not going anywhere!

The second step of harnessing inspiration is to link the vision with habits that lead to it. A great coach is curious about the work necessary to bring the vision closer. You ask questions that will create practical steps fuelled by what inspires the client.

The key is to discover positive motivation and convert it to positive habits.

Important—What Are the Priorities?

We make time for what is important to us. It's as simple as that. Our habits, actions, and behaviours will give us clues as to what our values are. What do we give our time to? Activities that hold purpose and meaning for us. What do we work at? We put effort into tasks that we prioritise. When we are engaged in activities that are not our priority or that do not lead to something of value to us, our energy is gradually drained. Our emotions will tell us when our values are trodden on. Frustration, anger, or sadness may indicate that we are no longer living according to our values.

A great coach asks questions to discover the client's values and then leads them to take steps to live in greater congruence with their values. (See the Values in Action exercise at the end of the chapter.) It is key to discover our values and live by them with intention and clarity because otherwise, we are pulled in many directions, living with confusion and lack of focus. Focus brings energy. Energy drives us forwards to success and achievement. Values bring the necessary focus, making decisions more effective. Values bring clear intention, leading to saving time and energy. Values highlight meaning and purpose, raising our motivation. In other words, when you know what you want to do, why you want to do it, and how you do it, you massively increase the chances of actually doing it! Without the harnessed energy of activated values, a vision remains a dream.

A great coach reveals the values that bring the client energy for the journey so that they can confidently move towards their goal. Harnessing this energy involves spending the necessary time to explore values, understand motivation, drill down to the core focus, and seek constant alignment with actions and reasons. The client's potential is increased when time is given to activities that are more likely to succeed. These activities are value-based and driven by the energy harnessed by living intentionally.

The key is to act from the focus of clear priorities.

Impact—The Difference It Makes

The impact of living out our vision and values is the difference it makes to our life and to the lives of those we influence. Impact indicates the effectiveness of our choices. We do not live in a vacuum, and we do not cultivate our vision and values as an abstract, theoretical amusement. We want our vision and values to make a difference. A deep human need is to make a difference, to be significant. So, the more impact our vision and values have, then the deeper our satisfaction and reward.

When we are aligned with our vision, we feel purpose. We know what we are here for. When we are aligned with our values, we feel meaning. We make sense of the journey. With habits and choices that support both vision and values, we feel joy! A great coach asks, "What is the impact on my well-being, my productivity, my progress, and my impact on others when I am running with my vision and values? Does it all flow?" If not, a great coach returns to what is important to them. Look again at what we do give our time to. And what brings us joy? I don't mean every day is all fluffy and sweet because there will be plenty of mundane days, some tough days, and a few days where we doubt it all. Mountain climbing demands a lot, but the peak is worth it. The serious climber with clear vision to reach the top will take into account the effort involved and declare it worth it.

"What's the point?" A cry often associated with despair and confusion is a very real question to ask simply to bring focus and motivation back. The point is our vision, which gives us purpose, and our values, which give meaning to the vision. To keep energised, it is necessary to witness discernible progress in the difference being made. A great coach will lead the client to think of ways to describe the impact. Keep a journal. Link an activity with the vision. Ask about the benefits along the way. What feedback is received from others? These pointers will act as nourishment on the journey towards the destination.

The key is to measure the difference made.

As a transformational coach, you are making a difference.

ACTIVITY

Values in Action

The purpose of this simple exercise is to affirm your values, to identify your values in day-to-day life and to take action in living more from the values. Living from our values brings more congruence, integrity, and joy.

- Using a list of values (I recommend Brené Brown's List of Values @brenebrown.com), ask your client to identify the values that are most important to them. To elicit values, ask a selection of the following questions:

What words resonate with you? What do you love to do? What is important to you? What do you want to build your life around? What are you passionate about? What brings you the deepest satisfaction or joy? How do you spend your time? What do you want to be remembered for? What do you fight for? What boosts your energy? What are your priorities in relationships? What do you most want to contribute?

- Aim to gather six to eight values that the client really affirms.
- Using that list, encourage the client to produce four statements. The client uses one value for statements 1 to 4. The exercise may be repeated as many times as necessary.

    1. I value ... [pick a value already identified above].
    2. I am ... [how I see my value in action].
    3. I want to ... [aspire to see more of my value in action].
    4. My action step is ... [take an action step based on the value].

For example:

1. I value connection.
2. I am connecting with my children intentionally every day on the school run.
3. I want to connect with my best friends more regularly.
4. My action step is to send a quick message every week to one friend.

1. I value adventure.
2. I am planning a trip to the mountains.
3. I want to take a course on windsurfing.
4. My action step is to research the top five schools in the area.

About the Author

Anna Prinz has been dedicated to people development her whole life—from humble beginnings of playing school with her little brother to gaining a teaching degree in English from Cambridge University. Anna has developed people in the UK, Tanzania, New Zealand, Egypt, and Lebanon. Anna lights up when connecting with others in the context of seeking wisdom. She is passionate about how to do life well and seeks to grow by remaining curious and digging deep.

Anna lives near London with her husband, three sons, and stepson. She loves candles by firelight, robins in her garden, and connecting with her boys around the dinner table.

Anna runs her coaching business, The Crossroads Coach, with a vision to support those at a crossroads in life, to bring clarity in decisions and joy in the journey.

Email: digdeepdreambig@gmail.com
Facebook: https://www.facebook.com/digdeepdreambig
LinkedIn: www.linkedin.com/in/anna-prinz-469831226
Blog: www.crossroadscoach.co.uk

CHAPTER 16

Vision-Centered Coaching: Guiding Clients to Discover their "Why"

By Mark Reinisch
Author of *The Wellness Ethic*, Life & Transformation Coach
Charleston, South Carolina

The two most important days in your life are the day you are born and the day you find out why.

—Mark Twain

The most successful lives are always fueled by purpose. Many of us know the inspiring, purpose-driven stories of Thomas Edison and his prolific inventions, Mahatma Gandhi and his nonviolent crusade to emancipate India, or Rosa Parks and her courageous resistance to segregation. But consider the dog shelter volunteer whose life purpose is to ease the suffering of animals. The hairdresser who is fulfilled by helping people feel beautiful. Or the devoted teacher who positively influences a thousand students during their career. These are all different lives, yet they share the common bond of the majestic nobility of a person embracing their mission in life.

Vision-Centered Coaching: Guiding Clients to Discover their "Why"

When you understand *why* you were born into this world—your life purpose—and act upon that life-affirming knowledge, positive energy flows throughout your being. You find joy and fulfillment in what you do. Work doesn't feel like "work." Instead, it's a vehicle to express the love inside you. Purpose becomes the nourishment that fuels your burning desire to get the most out of your existence by positively impacting the world.

When you are purpose-driven, you lean into your day with an intrinsic motivation that propels you forward in a direction congruent with your vision of a satisfying life—you are doing what you need to do to be happy and fulfilled. Purpose is why entrepreneurs work day and night to carve out market share in a competitive landscape. They *need* to bring their business ideas to life and provide for their family. It's why a parent with a full-time job may take on the daunting challenge of completing a college degree in the evenings and weekends. They *need* to move forward with their dreams and realize their full potential. Purpose fosters the requisite clarity, optimism, vitality, and resilience that is foundational to a meaningful life.

In a coaching relationship, when a coach and client explore life purpose, it can be a propellant that helps clients soar. A life purpose serves as the client's North Star. It provides a deeper understanding of what matters to them. It offers a bigger-picture perspective that steers clients away from becoming emotionally attached to annoyances and setbacks that will soon pass. When clients look at their circumstances through the lens of life purpose, they choose responses to life that honor their values and move them forward with their passions. Their life flows more smoothly as a result. They get better outcomes. They silence regrets.

You can facilitate a simple three-step process to help clients discover their life purpose. Here's a breakdown of the steps.

Discover Your Why

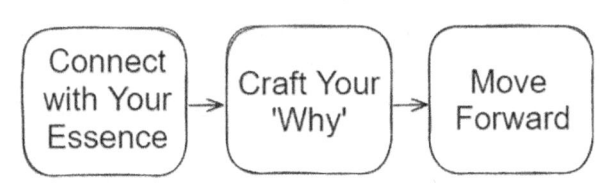

Connect with Your Essence → Craft Your 'Why' → Move Forward

Step 1: Connect with Your Essence

To discover your life purpose, you must be in touch with the essence of who you are. What are your values? Your passions? Your superpowers? The thread that connects the answers to those questions will lead you to your life purpose—what you were meant to do to be happy and fulfilled. Let's expand upon those three elements—values, passions, and superpowers—that help define who you are.

Your Values

The values you hold are the ideals that guide your conduct. What defines you when you're at your best? Your values can include character, teamwork, compassion, fairness, humility, family, equality, loyalty, excellence, personal growth, and more. A life that is on purpose promotes endless opportunities for a person's most cherished values to shine. For example, someone who values creativity and has a life purpose centered around using their creative talents to bring joy to themselves and others would be in their sweet spot if they activated their creative brain to write poetry at a café, teach a child how to paint, or solve a problem at work that required thinking out-of-the-box. Your values can provide clues to help you discover your life purpose. But there are more factors to consider. That brings us to your passions.

Your Passions

Another way to connect with your life purpose is to think about your passions—What do you love in your life? Then take it a step further—How would you rank in order what you love? I was first exposed to the concept of "ordered loves" in David Brooks' thought-provoking book *The Road to Character*. Ordered love refers to people having a pecking order of things they love. For instance, when you think about your career, supporting non-profits, financial security, family and friends, health, creative pursuits, travel, integrity, spirituality, and so on, how would you rank them in terms of what you love more?

Aligning your priorities and how you spend your time with your ordered loves—your passions—is essential to living a satisfying life. When you prioritize a lower love over a higher love, you have a disconnect that can degrade your spirit. Do you love being healthy but eat poorly or don't exercise regularly? Do you love your family but don't spend enough quality time with them? What gets in the way? Is it a lower love? When your life purpose and how you live your life are aligned with your higher loves, your everyday existence is in harmony with your spiritual essence. You thrive as a result.

Consider a person whose higher loves include family, helping others, and sports. They enjoy being active with their loved ones. They value how sports can promote teamwork, fitness, and sacrifice. They love coaching youth teams and helping children develop sports and life skills. Do you think there could be a fulfilling life purpose associated with a person's love of sports, family, and helping others? Most certainly.

As you think about your values and passions, you'll get closer to uncovering your life purpose. We'll add one more input to the mix to seal the deal: your superpowers.

Your Superpowers

Everyone is gifted at something. Everyone has superpowers. A person's superpowers could be used regularly, or they may have atrophied over time. They may even be undiscovered and waiting to be activated.

Thinking about your superpowers can inspire you to open your mind to the all-you-can-eat buffet of what you can accomplish when you apply your considerable talents to a worthy cause. For example, if you were passionate about improving the lives of others and had a superpower with carpentry, imagine what you could do when you combined those two interests: construct affordable, energy-efficient homes, volunteer your time to build a playground for a place of worship, or complete home improvement projects that will delight your family. We could come up with a hundred more ideas. Undoubtedly, there's a life purpose waiting to be discovered when you think about what someone could do if they had a gift for carpentry.

To identify your superpowers, examine what you've excelled at in your life, both personally and professionally, even during your childhood. If you asked those close to you, what would they suggest? Your superpowers could center around caregiving, strength and endurance, mechanics, analytics, intelligence, writing, programming, problem-solving, innovation, social networking, creativity, building things, leadership, and others. When you use your superpowers, you're engaged in life. You're flexing your mastery. You're doing exactly what you were created to do.

Now that you've sorted through your life purpose inputs, it's time to pull it together to craft your "why."

Step 2: Craft Your "Why"

A life purpose statement—your "why"—reflects how you want to live your life to impact the world. The statement should be personal and inspiring. It should align with your values, passions, and superpowers. It doesn't have to be earth-shaking. It can reflect the positive influence you want to have in your community, with your family, and even on yourself. You should choose a level of impact that will fulfill you.

A good litmus test for whether your life purpose statement captures your authentic "why" is envisioning being on your deathbed and looking back at your life. At that moment of truth, if you had lived your purpose throughout your days, would you be satisfied with your life? Would you have released the love inside of you? If so, your life purpose represents why you were born into this world. If not, then you have more reflection to do.

Though there is no standard format for a life purpose statement—you should use the style and format that resonates with you—I'll offer a simple framework that can get your creative juices flowing.

> **Life Purpose Statement**
>
> I <*what you do to impact the world*> through my <*how you do it*>.

Your values, passions, and superpowers inform *what you do* and *how you do it*. The following are examples of life purpose statements utilizing the framework:

- I exist to help young people realize their potential through my empathy, wisdom, and mentoring.
- I free animals from suffering through my compassion, activism, and leadership.
- I was born to make the world beautiful through my artistic talents.
- I bring justice to those in need through my tireless advocacy and legal expertise.
- I am devoted to saving our planet for future generations by doing my part and leading others to do the same.
- I inspire the world to grow spiritually through my gift of storytelling.

You may have noticed that these life purpose statements don't detail exactly what a person does to achieve their purpose; instead, they provide a theme for one's life. They point in a general direction, mainly in the person's control. The statements recognize that there are many ways to live a life on purpose.

Consider the life purpose statement: *I exist to help young people realize their full potential through my empathy, wisdom, and mentoring.* It sounds like the life purpose statement of a teacher, right? It could be. But it also could describe a parent, a daycare provider, a mentor, a community volunteer, a blogger, a youth minister, a coach, a philanthropist, and hundreds of other endeavors. I recommend keeping your life purpose statements at the thematic level to give yourself ample room to explore your purpose in diverse and inspired ways throughout your life.

The following *Discover Your Life Purpose* worksheet can help you develop your life purpose statement:

Discover Your Life Purpose	
Values	**Your Top 5**
○ Accountability ○ Achievement ○ Adventure ○ Authenticity ○ Balance ○ Belonging ○ Challenge ○ Character, Honor, & Integrity ○ Commitment ○ Compassion ○ Competence ○ Creativity ○ Curiosity ○ Discipline & Order ○ Diversity, Inclusion, & Equality ○ Empathy ○ Empowerment ○ Excellence ○ Faith ○ Family & Friends ○ Flexibility ○ Freedom ○ Fun ○ Grace ○ Gratitude ○ Growth ○ Happiness ○ Health & Wellness ○ Hope ○ Humility ○ Humor ○ Imagination ○ Individuality ○ Influence ○ Inspiration ○ Intuition ○ Justice ○ Kindness ○ Learning ○ Leadership ○ Love ○ Loyalty ○ Mastery ○ Meaning & Purpose ○ Optimism ○ Patience ○ Peace ○ Pleasure ○ Prosperity ○ Quality ○ Resilience ○ Responsibility ○ Sacrifice ○ Safety & Security ○ Self-esteem & Self-respect ○ Service & Generosity ○ Simplicity ○ Spirituality ○ Stability ○ Surrender ○ Wisdom ○ <other values>…	
Ordered Loves	**Your Top 5**
○ Adventure ○ Animals ○ Art ○ Charity ○ Family & Friends ○ Food ○ Health ○ Hobbies ○ Independence ○ Integrity/Character ○ Learning ○ Leisure ○ Money ○ Music ○ Nature ○ Professional Accomplishment ○ Recreation ○ Reputation ○ Safety ○ Security ○ Spirituality ○ Sports ○ Technology ○ Travel ○ <other loves>…	

Superpowers	Your Top 4
○ Adapting to Change ○ Analytics ○ Architecting ○ Building Things ○ Caregiving ○ Creativity ○ Critical Thinking ○ Design ○ Emotional Intelligence ○ Empathy ○ Energy ○ Engineering ○ Finance & Money Management ○ Humor ○ Innovation ○ Inspiration ○ Intelligence ○ Learning Languages ○ Leadership ○ Making Friends ○ Mechanics ○ Memory ○ Music ○ Networking ○ Persuasion ○ Problem Solving ○ Programming ○ Self-control ○ Service ○ Speaking ○ Spirituality ○ Sports ○ Systems Thinking ○ Teaching ○ Technology ○ Time Management ○ Vision ○ Wisdom ○ Writing ○ <other superpowers>...	
Your Life Purpose Statement	

Celebrate your accomplishment once you've crafted a life purpose statement that inspires you. It can transform your life. That is, provided you put it into action. That leads us to Step 3: Move Forward.

Step 3: Move Forward

To transition your life purpose from concept to reality, you can assess how the critical aspects of your life support your life purpose. Those insights will help you determine what you should start, stop, or continue doing to make your purpose come alive. We'll run through a case study to illustrate how that could be done.

Stella, mid-40s, is married and with two children, ages 16 and 18. She is a corporate attorney from humble beginnings and was the first person in her family to attend college. She is grateful for the work ethic her parents instilled in her, the sacrifices they made, and the mentoring her teachers provided. She knows from experience that young people need a nurturing environment to be successful.

When considering her life purpose, she started with her values and identified family, education, and equality as the most important. When she developed a list of her ordered loves, her top love was her family, followed by healthy living, giving back, learning, and professional achievement. Her analytical mind, leadership, and empathy were her superpowers.

When she created her life purpose statement, she came up with the following: *I dedicate my life to helping people live their dreams, including my family and myself, through my leadership and devotion to personal development.* This vision brought a smile to her face. She knew it was what she was meant to do.

Now, she had to make it real in all the relevant aspects of her life. She first examined her career. Was she pursuing her dreams and making the impact that she expected? She liked being a lawyer but wasn't inspired by being a corporate attorney. Was there another type of law she could practice that better aligned with her life purpose? Perhaps serving as a lawyer for a non-profit? Would she enjoy stepping out of her legal role and leading a non-profit that served disadvantaged children? Or at least volunteer her time and offer pro bono legal expertise? She knew supporting non-profits aligned with her purpose in life. She committed to developing a plan to move in that direction.

She then turned her attention to her family. How could her family align with her life purpose? She always thought she was a supportive wife and mother. But did she ever ask them what their dreams were and whether they were getting all the support they needed from her? Not really. When she discussed the topic with her husband, he suggested she lead their family through an exercise to develop their life purpose statements. She loved the idea. It would inspire them to get excited about living their dreams while giving her insights on how she could support their pursuits.

Stella paused and reflected. She had filled a couple of pages in her notebook with possibilities that thrilled her. She knew she had to complete much more discovery and then prioritize her focus and develop a plan. She also understood that she would have to say no to activities misaligned to her life purpose, so she could say yes to interests that stirred her spirit. But what a wonderful problem to have—an abundance of opportunities that would bring love into her life and the universe.

When life coaches help clients develop their life purpose and put it into action, the clients are positioned to live a life spiritually engineered to manifest love and satisfaction.

> Purpose is indispensable to a successful life:
> We were meant to love our life purpose and live it every day.

ACTIVITY

See Discover Your Life Purpose within the chapter.

About the Author

Mark Reinisch is an author, life coach, and transformation leader who specializes in helping people move forward in the direction of their dreams. Mark has decades of executive experience leading business transformation in corporate America. As side hustles, he founded a social media startup, shepherded it to a successful buyout, and has written a dozen comedic screenplays. His current book project—*The Wellness Ethic*, a self-help book that makes wellness accessible and actionable (and entertaining!)—is scheduled for release in 2024.

Email: WellnessEthic@gmail.com
Website: www.WellnessEthic.com

CHAPTER 17

Coaching Creatively: Giving Voice to Confidence

By Marisol Rodriguez
Creative Leadership Coach and Facilitator
Chicago, Illinois

Curiosity's reason for existing is not simply to be a tool for acquiring knowledge; it reminds us that we're alive.

—Brené Brown

In 2017, I was at a crossroads in my career. I had spent the past three years learning innovation tools and methods at a financial firm where I felt like an outsider. I loved everything I was exposed to about growth mindset and creativity, yet I wanted more. It all seemed surface level, and I wanted to explore how people create change at a deeper level. In my nine years at the company, its cold and unemotional environment felt like the antithesis to how I wanted to work compared to my previous career as an advocate for victims of sexual assault and violence, where I delivered training to first responders on how to provide more empathetic care.

While I longed for deeper conversation, I wanted to avoid trauma work and instead help others by moving toward a more hopeful future where they could take empowered action. I remember enjoying lunch with a mentor one day, confiding that I wanted something more out of my career to help others more powerfully. And her response was, "Have you ever thought about coaching?" For me, this was a true light-bulb moment in my life. It felt like the heavens were singing the more she described the coaching process. Everything that was wilting inside of me suddenly came alive, like a flower unfolding, stretching itself to bask in the warmth of the sun. My offerings to you in this chapter are the key tools and gifts that have informed my coaching work since that pivotal moment and that help me go deeper with my clients to co-create a strengthened ability to alchemize fear into courageous action.

Your Intuition Is a Gift

Your intuition is your guidance system in a chaotic, complex world, and it is the KEY gift that will empower you to stretch yourself into a perceptive and brave coach. The small intuitive hits we receive; that small voice that pokes at us to pause and question our client when they say something that seems off or dissonant—Don't ignore that voice! Don't discount that niggle, the (oftentimes) whisper that there's something not being said. Too often we avoid our gut instinct to step into brave and powerful coaching. It's important to air out these small intuitions and check in with your client to see if they resonate.

A client was recently recounting her frustration with her company. She felt pressure to prove her value in her role and to climb the corporate ladder. But for her, that striving was empty. She instead wanted to focus on continuing to provide solid service to her clients who were often the underdogs within the industry. This was work she had done well for 20 years: developing strong relationships and building trust.

In the call, my eyes were drawn to a piece of artwork in a back window. It appeared as if a child had made it, but it was bright and beautiful, taking in the sun. My intuition nagged at me to ask about it and pull her out of this negative space. And so I did, and her look of shocked surprise piqued my curiosity. She had placed it there to be a visual reminder of her mother's role in her life, and I was the first to ever bring attention to it. Her mother had passed a year or two prior and had made it during the height of her dementia. My client cherished this piece because it highlighted her mother's artistry, even in illness. She savored her mother's memory and became overwhelmed with emotion as she described the lessons she imparted.

I asked, "What would your mother say to you now about this situation?" And with a look of amusement, she shared that her mother's life was focused on the creation of connection through art, music, and play. And that she would remind her to make music with her work and to stay creative, strong, and deeply engaged with those around her from a place of joy. It opened a door to possibilities and gave her renewed awareness that somewhere along the way, she had disengaged from her colleagues.

She decided to start personally connecting to her network again, to open the door for new relationships, connections, and service. Within seven months, she was promoted. I like to think that something was unlocked; her perspective was shifted that day. Had I not listened to that nagging intuition, perhaps she wouldn't have reached this place of insight.

Remember that coaching can be playful. Call out what you see in the room. Use the space around you. Use metaphor, art, song, images, etc., to powerfully awaken a client's imagination and spark emotion. Are you stretching your creativity as a coach? Are you incorporating play? In your next client call, push yourself to use metaphor to weave a story. What are the metaphors you often use? Take the client out of the problem they're in and help them see the world through new vantage points.

Do they have a view of a river? Use it.

Ask them to describe it. What is the function of a river? If they were to look at their situation through the lessons conveyed in the flowing of a river, what would they be? Watch them reveal how the movement of a river reminds them of the movement of life—the value of going with the flow and swiftly overcoming obstacles that might be in their way. This helps to highlight <u>how</u> they are living rather than on <u>what</u> they are experiencing.

Has your client just sighed heavily at a comment they made or question you posed? Ask them about it. "Tell me what that is. What are you carrying in that sigh?" This is all information for your intuition to explore from a place of curiosity. Follow it. Call it out. And watch the magic that unfolds.

Separating From Fear

Your clients want to be seen, understood, validated, and to feel alive. They want to be championed, challenged, and encouraged toward their goals while feeling held and supported by you. Their fear will always be the loudest voice they'll hear—are you coaching their fear or their groundedness? Here's how to tell the difference.

The voice of fear is repetitive. It focuses on the problem or areas of lack and speaks in an anxious tone. It only sees the "black and white" of a situation—"Is this possible? Yes or no. Am I qualified? Yes or no." It has no need for evidence and makes proclamations from a place of self-critique.

Your job is to move your client out of this place and foster the connection they have to their realistic, confident thinking voice. That voice is always curious and wants to gather evidence to inform conclusions. It's able to deal with complexity and the gray areas. It asks open-ended questions: "How might this be possible?" It's forward moving, seeks solutions, and is calm in the face of difficulty. This is the self-supportive voice. The voice that fully embodies the popular idiom used in the improv world, "Yes, and …"

As you start a coaching relationship, one of the first things you might consider doing with your client is to help them personify the voice of fear. Help them connect the dots between how they are being and how that might get in the way of what they want to be doing. Have them describe this part of themselves, their inner critic, with great detail: the name, style of clothing, place of residence, relationships, hobbies, repeated sayings, etc. The goal is to bring this aspect of themselves to life as a separate entity.

Instruct them to write a letter of separation to their critic. This is a letter that will free them from this voice of control as it pertains to their decision making. Have the client read aloud to you what they've written, which is a powerful way for them to embrace and claim the changes they're committed to making. As homework, they can also find someone to read this to, someone who will respect the activity, will not laugh, and may also benefit from doing it themselves. This will create accountability for your client. Saying it out loud holds power and provides a witness to what they want. This is key to landing the impact of this exercise.

Guided Visualizations

Mindfulness is a powerful tool to help calm a client's activated nervous system and give them access to their internal clarity, which I learned through my Co-Active training. Guided visualizations can bring this clarity to life by personifying this voice as their inner leader. You can help calm their nervous system through simple breathing exercises and a body scan. Have them close their eyes, take three deep centering breaths, and sit comfortably while relaxing their body from the top of the head to the tips of their toes. In a calming voice, tell them: "Relax your face, shoulders, and all tension moving down your arms. Releasing any stress out the tips of your fingers, letting go of tension in your stomach. Relaxing your legs, knees, and releasing down, down, down out through the tips of your toes."

Ask your client to tap into their imagination and to picture a place that they can completely make up in their mind that is their safe space. The point is to be fully present, safe, and connected to this space of beauty and contentment. Have all five of their senses tapped into this visualization. Instruct them to take in the details. Are there birds chirping, the scent of grass or water in the air? Is there warmth here? Are the colors vibrant? Can they feel grains of sand on their feet? Whatever it is, their senses can make the space around them come alive. Get creative and come up with the questions and prompts that might bring them further into the visualization.

You are guiding your client to tap into safety, helping them to calm their nervous system. And you can then tell them that in this safe haven, they can meet the part of themselves that is always calm, courageous, loving, and confident: their inner wise, compassionate self that has clarity, strength, and an infinite heart. Have this part of themselves come into view from far away at first, walking toward them, eager to meet them with a sense of excitement in the air. This is their inner authority and guide. Give them time to meet this part of themselves and to be in conversation. To ask this part of themselves what they should know about their life and what is possible for their journey ahead. You can guide your client to imagine receiving something from their authority with a message. A gift that will guide them through challenges. Give the client time to receive and listen for any guidance they receive in silence.

Trust your client to get there. Allowing time (at least 15-20 minutes) for quiet space and to be immersed in the visioning exercise. You can slowly bring them back to their body, instructing them to take deep breaths again, and upon opening their eyes, to take notes in silence about their experience. Writing down what they want to remember before verbally having them share this with you.

I've also used visioning to help clients grappling between two decisions. Always starting with closing their eyes, taking deep breaths to connect to their body, and asking them to consider one option and notice if they feel expansive and open, or if they feel constricted, fearful, or closed off somehow. And repeat this exercise with the second option. Often, clients will notice they are drawn to one over the other and can feel more confident in their decision making using this as a test for what feels right.

There's Power in Your Voice

Your client's voice is powerful. Have them use it. Give them opportunities to read and share aloud with you, as well as others in their life. If you've not discovered the work of Luvvie Ajayi Jones, I would encourage you to pick up her book, *Professional Troublemaker: The Fear-Fighter Manual*. In it, she describes how to write up an Oríkì, or "your personal hype mantra." Essentially, it's a self-affirming mantra or proclamation of who you are. This is an exercise to throw away all humility and acknowledge what makes you proud. It's a claiming of your superpowers. Remember the show *Game of Thrones*? When they introduce the character of Daenerys, they say, "*Daenerys Stormborn of the House Targaryen. First of Her Name. The Un-burnt. Queen of the Andals and the First Men. Khaleesi of the Great Grass Sea. Breaker of Chains. Mother of Dragons.*" Now THAT is a powerful Oríkì.

I tried this with a client who was often speaking negatively about himself. He would downplay his abilities. As homework, I assigned him the task of writing his own Oríkì and following the formula that Luvvie lays out: "[First name and Middle name] of house [Last name] [Number of his/her/their name, i.e., Juniors are second of their name] [Noun: occupation or description] of [Noun: thing]". Here's an example I created for myself:

"Marisol of House Rodriguez
First of her name
A quiet poet of joy
Queen Empress at the birth of her daughters
Conscious creator of her life story
Puerto Rican seeker of truth
Healer and coach
Illuminator of powerful memories resurfaced
A song that awakens the soul"

I hope you can feel the significance of this mantra. It's an exercise to own my personal strengths. When I asked my client to read his to me aloud, he could barely get through it. Through his tears and with a shaky voice, he claimed his name, his history, the legacy from his father. He articulated the pride he felt for his story. It was a powerful thing for him to declare verbally. To own his journey and his unique gifts. It helped him to step into gratitude for the challenges he faced and to embrace how he'd owned the legacy he built for himself. It's what was needed to have him live a more purposeful and intentional life moving forward. Owning this part of himself and knowing that it informed the possibilities that lay in wait. Try it out and see what unfolds.

You might also consider having your client write up an acceptance speech to thank themselves for how far they've gotten to where they are in life. Have you ever heard Snoop Dogg's speech thanking himself when receiving his Hollywood star on the Walk of Fame? It's truly inspiring and a certain confidence boost. They can begin each sentence with: "I want to thank me for …" and list at least seven things to acknowledge. Ask them to read it to you from the heart and with conviction and watch them take up space in the room.

Coaching Is Not a Formula

To close, I advise you not to follow a formula. Specific coaching tools and skills are but one tool in your toolbox. It is your life experience, your expertise, your voice, your unique perspective that will flavor your coaching.

Do not discount those gifts and play small. Do not play into mimicking another person's approach.

Find your own style of coaching that sets you apart from the pack. Your clients are paying for the unique experience of you and your gifts. Imagine if you only follow a formula you've been given and decide to create the right "steps" to the process that's identical for each client. How rigid would that feel? It lacks spontaneous creation. All the heart will be taken out of the coaching conversation.

Staying connected to your heart is key to powerful coaching. Coaching from the heart center is a powerful tool for shifting your client into inspired action. This is not about centering you in their story. It is not about taking over their narrative. It's about championing your client, breathing life into their dreams, and encouraging them to move forward with confident action even in the face of fear. You are playing a special role in their life. You are godsent. Embrace this role and remember to own your energy fully as a coach to facilitate the transformation your clients are seeking.

Godspeed.

ACTIVITY

See the Oríkì Formula, visioning, and letter of separation activity within the chapter.

About the Author

Marisol Rodriguez is a Certified Professional Co-Active Coach and Innovation Lab Facilitator at a derivatives exchange where she has served for over a decade. Marisol relishes the opportunity to assist individuals and teams to gain clarity about their goals and improve their ability to collaborate in complex environments. She teaches leaders how to quiet the noise of "productivity for productivity's sake" and has a sharpened ability to pinpoint the behaviors that get in the way of success.

As a professional coach, Marisol uses her experience in crisis intervention for victims of domestic violence and sexual assault—to bring compassion and heart to her client work. She combines mindfulness, intuition, and her experience in innovation frameworks to shift people out of problem-based thinking and into solution-based mindsets. Her deeply empathetic approach marries creativity and ideation to help clients navigate challenges and enhance their leadership abilities.

Website: www.awakentolifecoach.com
Email: marisol@awakentolifecoach.com
LinkedIn: https://www.linkedin.com/in/marisol-rodriguez1/
YouTube: http://Awakentolife.me/chb or @marisolrodriguezlife

CHAPTER 18

Marriage Coaching

By Alisa A. Sanè
CEO & Founder of 90 Day Health and Life Coach, Author
Arlington, Tennessee

Introduction to the Marriage Coach

Writing about a topic that increases success in communication, intimacy, respect, and a lifelong desire to work cohesively with a partner is always a pleasure. I find joy knowing that broken relationships can be healed. As a life coach, when dealing with difficult marriages, one thing is for sure: Marriage coaching is different other forms. It is responsible for untangling the frequent stresses of a failing union and for bringing the relationship back into alignment.

Let's briefly define this system of cultivating a marriage between two people who have decided to marry but who might come from two different world views, upbringings, values, and maybe even cultures and religions.

What Is Marriage Coaching?

As a marriage coach, when assessing clients who choose to work with me, I describe it as focus-driven, goal-directed momentum that moves couples forward by dealing with past problems swiftly. I don't necessarily ponder over the past as they have encapsulated the marriage, but by naming the problem areas from the past and pushing forward with strategies that will give the union a new voice, great things can happen.

As you begin reading this chapter, think of this form of marriage coaching as a deliverable to guide many areas in people's lives. While reading this chapter, the reader may find themselves or see their own relationship in the chapter. The reader might also see their coaching client's situation. The goal in marriage coaching is to understand the desire to push forward and heal the present wounds of a marriage and help things start to make sense again. This can lead toward a path forward to discover answers to much-needed questions to assist in halting the disease that has infected a once peaceful union.

A good marriage coach's strategy that could be presented when working with a couple often centers around the development of a personal policy for a marriage. In this policy, the team will define the issues that are currently present, measurable, and solvable. The marriage policy can be a one-pager. It doesn't need to be lengthy. The marriage policy is personally designed and is crucial to follow to move the couple forward. As a couple dealing with marriage woes, keep in mind that if you are not moving forward in your marriage, you are either stuck or moving backward.

Another primary focus of marriage coaching is post-marriage coaching. This is when a couple has completed the set number of sessions with a good coach and has moved to living life without the marriage coach's physical and emotional support. Couples can breathe a sigh of relief that a great coach is always a text, email, or phone call away if they encounter bumps in their relationship, especially if those issues that brought them into marriage coaching rear their ugly heads again.

Often, after marriage coaching sessions are completed, one person in the marriage may return to their previous behaviors because it appears comfortable. As a marriage coach, I caution couples not to slip back into old behaviors that can end their marriage in divorce.

Marriage coaching has goals and focuses similar to those in marriage counseling therapy. Some of the skills used by coaches and counselors may be transferable. Even still, I always keep the premise in mind that I work in the present with a couple and not necessarily dwell in the past (as can happen in therapy).

I often use individual life coaching sessions with my couples to work on personal or professional issues that have also played a negative role in the marriage and have created areas of concern. Most clients who seek coaching, in particular, want to flourish, make dreams come true, and live fully. This is also a focus of marriage coaching. The clients' best marriage forward is all within the couple's framework. One of the main principles when working with couples is ensuring the clients are not checked out of the relationship. As the spouse who initiated the marriage coaching sessions, it may be exhausting to try to reel in the spouse who is fed up or checked out. For a failing marriage to get back on track again, it is important to get both individuals in the relationship back in alignment. I mention this carefully only to say that my ideal client as a marriage coach is working with a couple who wants to save their marriage and doesn't feel too much contempt for their spouse. Rather, they realize there are some problem areas that can be fixed. They see a path forward to better their marriage and eliminate the adverse effects of the issues.

From the very start of marriage coaching, assessment through observation, body language, and spoken words are ways I have learned to allow the best couples to guide their positive conclusions for solutions in their marriage.

When a couple is assessed, detailed, and presented with a better path forward, continued coaching sessions, combined with goal-directed activities, create better outcomes for the marriage. It should be noted that these clients have worked hard and can get back on track if they want to.

As a marriage coach, I often make initial contact by conducting telephone consultations, which usually last for 15 minutes and are also free of charge. This is when I make sure to check for the right fit between coach and client. I schedule the marriage coaching session with both individuals at the same time. In the second session, I split the couple into individual sessions to better understand how they may view the current issues they are dealing with differently or the same. Then, I bring the couple together in a third session to dive deeper into their concerns. I may suggest books and workbooks that closely align with their current issues as they can work on these together and look to them for guidance and reference.

If the couple also has parenting concerns, I will suggest books centered around boundaries with children. Some clients I have encountered struggle with this area as well because, again, being raised in different homes, there can be challenges of how one parent may want to discipline or praise children. It may be in conflict with the other spouse's agency, but for a successful marriage, these issues must be addressed.

In the end, being a marriage coach is one of the most rewarding things I can imaging because I get to participate in the reconstruction of a union between broken individuals. With both a clear strategy and a true sense of caring, even very troubled marriages have hope, and as a marriage coach, I am honored to be part of that.

ACTIVITY

For Couples Who Seek to Solve Marriage Woes

I spoke of a marriage policy for couples in marriage coaching. Let me expound on this a bit. I will define a policy as how I see it to fit the average couple I've encountered during my coaching. Of course, this is only a suggestion and shouldn't be misconstrued to guarantee success. Each marriage policy will be different.

The Marriage Policy

The marriage policy is basically a set of written terms which the individuals in the marriage agree with as areas of conduct. When developing a marriage policy, the couple should always look at the action plan they are growing as a course to live by. Remember that nothing is written in stone and cannot be tweaked when future problems arise.

To create the marriage policy, the first thing that needs to be done is the couple must decide on a time, place, and forward action goals to stimulate positive change.

As a couple dives into this exercise, make sure there's no distraction. Try to draw a rough draft of how you see your recipe for a soundproof marriage policy that would lead the couple in the right direction. The couple can think of it as an outline of their present life, writing down all current issues that need to be addressed. These issues can be tailored to better fit the marriage they want. They are writing out what marriage would look good to them at this stage.

As the couple develops their policy, they should always keep in mind to give each other grace. The plan should adopt a simple but complex practice for couples to follow to be best for each other amid distress. This positive focus helps the couple with an unconditional positive regard. The marriage policy should reject the judgment of the couple and should adopt available tools the couple has to move forward with.

Once the policy is fully developed with goals and tools and are obtainable and reachable, the couple can do something straightforward. They can type it up and keep it visible in their home, and as a marriage coach, I would even suggest making the marriage policy accessible on their devices, such as phones or tablets. This may seem silly, but you could think of the old saying, "Out of sight, out of mind." If you don't routinely visit the policy, the couple may forget its purpose and rules for their marriage. However, if both individuals in the marriage are dedicated to reminding themselves of the marriage policy and its terms, there is a great chance that the couple can succeed in rebuilding the relationship to a positive place of love and acceptance.

About the Author

Alisa A. Sanè is the author of *Dirty Housewife*. She was born in Cleveland, Ohio, and lived there for 38 years before moving to Arlington, Tennessee. A lover of words since she was a teenager, she has been writing for over 30 years. She wrote *Dirty Housewife* for her understanding of loving her husband, Moussa, intensely. The *Dirty Housewife* will be released on Amazon in 2024.

Alisa lives to laugh with good friends, spends time with her fantastic daughter, and writes fiction endlessly. You can find her hanging out in a coffee house, drinking black tea, or people-watching, creating stories. She graduated with a BA in Social Work from Cleveland State University and a Master of Art in Adult Education and Education & Training from the University of Phoenix. She is a certified Christian marriage and relationship coach and a certified life and health coach.

Alisa is the Founder and CEO of 90 Day Health & Life Coach LLC and The Marriage Coach School, which offers online classes where singles or couples can learn skills to enhance their marriage. 90 Day Health & Life Coach LLC also provides a home study course or telehealth to become a certified coach with dedicated topics specially developed to a desired coach's niche. 90 Day Health and Life Coach is located in Arlington, Tennessee, and is open 24 hours to sign up and complete the course online.

Email: alisa@90dayhealthandlifecoach.com
Website: 90dayhealthandlifecoach.com
Facebook: facebook.com/90dayhealthandlifecoach.com
Instagram: @90dayhealthnlifecoach.com
LinkedIn: www.linkedin.com/in/alisa-sane608b07188

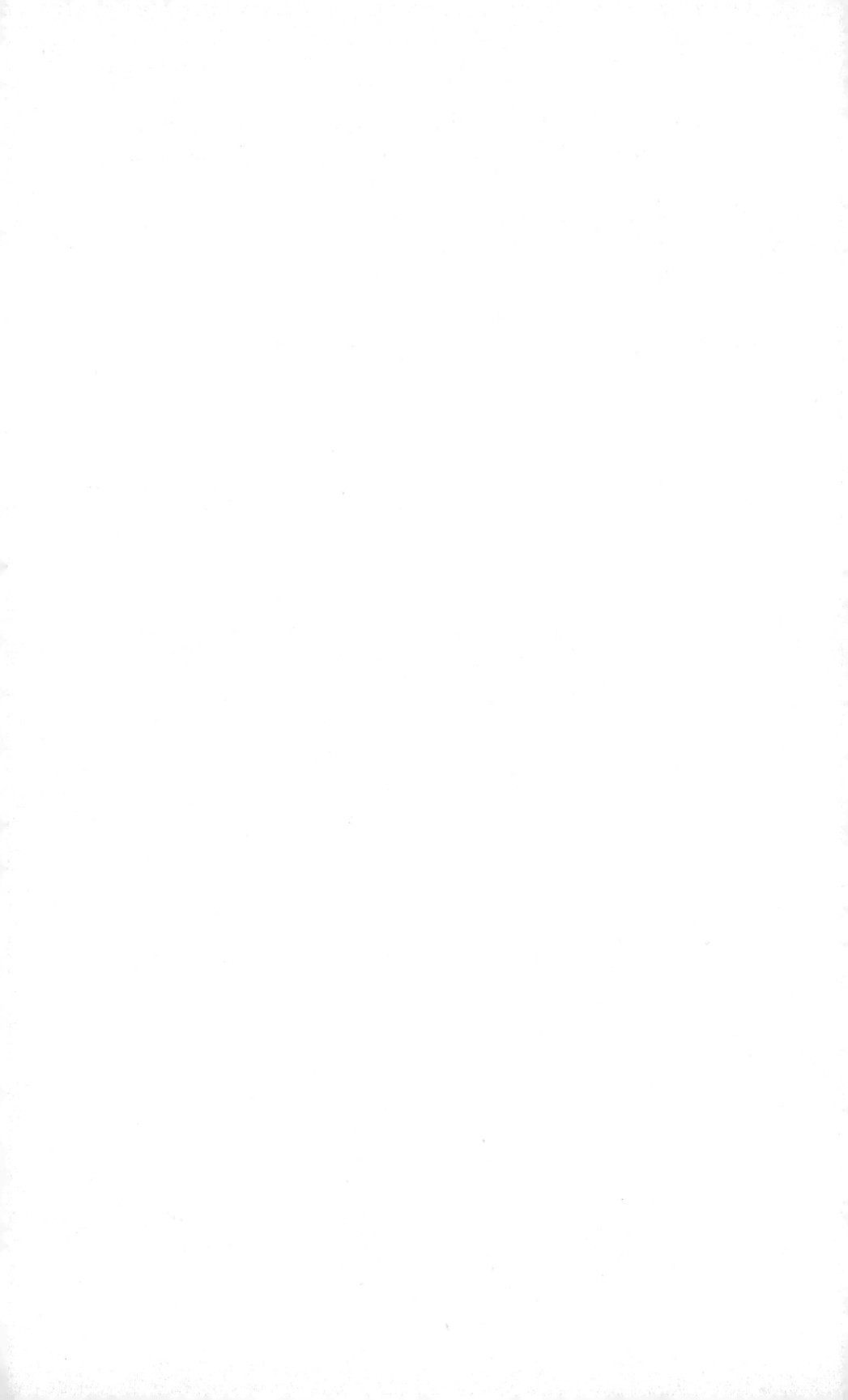

CHAPTER 19

Leading with Love

By Ya'ara Segal, CPCC
Life Coach & Trainer for Social Impact
Zurich, Switzerland

*Have enough courage to trust love one more
time and always one more time.*

—Maya Angelou

Love—It lived within us all since before we were born. Its virtues are felt in each step we take. By learning to intentionally utilize it as our contact point with the world, we get to open more hearts and courageously help people move forward.

Love goes where needed, being the powerful force she is. As the leader, it is the coach who would be admirably serving their coachee by insisting and preserving the loving force alive in the coaching sphere. It starts with clearing background noises and only speaking truths. Truth is the language of love. Words of truth are louder than any voice. To speak the truth in spite of the pain it conflicts is bravery. To stay with the pain is fierceness. The traits of a loving coach.

Introduction

Setting the Stage: The Power of Love in Coaching

In this chapter, we embark on a journey to explore the profound impact of leading with love in the world of coaching. Love is a transformative force that creates a deep connection between coach and coachee, while fostering personal growth and development. As we delve into this topic, you'll discover the practical application of love in coaching, from preparation of the individual process to the organizational coaching sphere.

The Coaching Journey: Personal Transformation Through Love

Seeing one's greatness and delicately pulling its strings. Trusting oh so many sorts of greatness to unfold. That's the coach's movement, regardless of the coaching model we follow. We pursue fragments of thoughts, hints of ideas, and elusive feelings. Relentlessly accommodating the space and our movement to the accurate forms the coachee, the human we hold presents each session.

The coach's commitment to another person's becoming process translates to a moral command to extend free love. Many know how to love yet are not necessarily trained in instilling love as a coaching practice.

It is our responsibility and privilege to demonstrate love in our actions. Otherwise, we will be neglecting our coachee's most basic needs from fully coming to light. Regardless of our physical attributes, socialization, and life circumstances, we all share the simple need to be loved. Psychsociological research keeps proving how profoundly love and the lack of it affect us. From building the foundation of our being in our infant years until serving as a driving force and also as a savior and rescue during our life in times of adversity.

When we are successful in leading with love, we honor values of authenticity and openness and allow wholeness to unfold.

Imagine one of your coachees. Keep them in your mind's eye while absorbing this definition of love by American author, scholar, and activist Bell Hooks: "The will to extend one's self for the purpose of nurturing one's own or another's spiritual growth. Love is as love does. Love is an act of will—namely, both an intention and an action."

To illustrate the impact love had on my coaching, let me share my experience with Shira. I must admit that initially, I didn't particularly like Shira. It's essential to acknowledge that not all coaching relationships start with an immediate connection. Yet as I wholeheartedly embraced the principles of love in coaching, I underwent a significant transformation. My energy, my approach, and the entire dynamic of coaching Shira evolved in ways I couldn't have anticipated. I chose to love her anew every coaching session. Before the Zoom camera turned on, I reflected on her virtues. When one of her reactions triggered an irritation within me, I dug deeper and found something I value. I explored and cleared up assumptions I might have that are standing in our way. I named them and found their source within me. I have cleaned my heart.

When referring to love as an act, rather than a feeling, Bell Hooks accurately describes the intention of applying our skills and knowledge to support our coachees in nurturing themselves, tapping into their strengths, and expanding. It is the loving movement between us that encourages development.

A conscious decision to lead from love gradually creates a powerful impact—open hearts. Crafting the skill will allow love to become your coaching default mode.

Practices–Crafting a Nourishing Movement

Even in the most humanistic of educational systems, love is confined to literature or art classes, and its practices aren't explicitly thought about.

For the majority of Western society's professionals across the different industry fields, staying correct is the comfortable base of operation. Correct means emotionless. Love finds itself waiting outside locked office doors. Allowed to participate in our lives as an afternoon activity.

As coaching is associated with professional development, we can easily forget that our work would be partially effective and temporary lasting without consciously inviting love to our coaching partnership.

People search for coaching support because they wish to overcome a hurdle, move on to the next step, or get unstuck. The aims are very practical and important, yet those are the surface-level reasons. Their real need is to see themselves and to be seen as who they really are, to know that they are enough. They are searching for help in exposing the person they are behind their degrees and job titles. To get to know that person and love them. An intentionally loving coach is able to notice and explore the different levels of the whole human being. Hence, loving support goes far beyond realizing their next step to realizing their desired life movement.

Coaching provides a person with an opportunity to deepen self-learning and move forward. When hearts are open, the exploration possibilities go deeper and wider. Even coaches who naturally embrace the loving movement would benefit from gaining mindful practices.

Terminology matters here. Using the word "love," with all its associations, holds us accountable for making sure that the coaching space we create is absorbed with care, compassion, and complete honesty.

Preparation: Setting the Loving Foundation

Pre-Coaching Rituals: Cultivating Love Before the Session

It is possible and valuable to isolate love's valuable and possible manifestations the coach can initiate within the coaching sphere.

Our coaching tools remain almost unchanged. Yet by provoking love, their effect will be meaningful and lasting.

Even one or two minutes of pre-session reflection can support a valuable tuning in toward the human you are about to meet. You might not be able to come up with too many descriptions. Yet even a mere few will lead you toward the desired beneficial mindset. Before your meeting, take a few minutes to reflect on:

- All that is beautiful in the person you are about to see
- All that matters to them
- All they are longing for
- All of your offerings that will serve them best

During the Coaching Session: Practicing Love

Active Listening with Love: A Key to Effective Coaching

As always in coaching, active listening stays key. The coach remains open, curious, and non-judgmental since we are there in the service of our coachee's stretching soul. In addition to that, we have opportunities during the course of the session to fold loving messages in the form of questions or short acknowledgments, which will support softening and widening the state of mind. The coaching mutual dance is the opportunity to plant the seeds that will later bloom.

Embracing Complexity: Love Can Be Found in Deep Exploration

Full awareness and reflection of everything that is beautiful, powerful, and meaningful. Tiny as you might feel the clue is, stay curious about all that can be revealed. The coach always holds an imaginary flashlight. Shedding light has a marvelous encouraging effect. It could very well be that your coachee doesn't notice or isn't able to see some important pieces. Metaphorical hugs in the form of heartfelt acknowledgments enhance engagement levels. Missing out on hugging opportunities can unintentionally make your coachee feel like they have been kicked.

A Clear Voice: Creating a Noise-Cancelling Effect

Your coachee probably has so much distracting noise in their life. Your session is an opportunity for them to explore, hear, play with all the voices, and single out the ones that inspire them, that they truly believe and wish to align with. When present, love can do a lot to balance and positively tilt that weight. Love has a voice of its own that is a mighty counter energy against the forces of negative self-evaluation. Your words are drops of water, carving slowly though the stone.

Speak the Truth, They'll Listen

A loving base point only enhances our obligation to the truth. Yes, we see the best there is, and at the same breath, we are there to lovingly ask hard questions. In this case, loving means we are brave enough to ask and trust that our coachee has the courage to face it. A loving coach feels how they should dose the truth confrontation according to the indication they receive from the coachee. According to the readiness level and a bit above. A loving coach holds and believes the full life can exist for their coachee and strives to dig deep in case there isn't an alignment, even if all seemingly relevant things are addressed.

A great example would be Tamara, a lovely coachee with whom I worked with a few years ago. Tamara was in the early stages of building her new professional path. Forty minutes into the session, when we were almost summarizing, I felt we had to stop. Tamara was confidently discussing the position she was about to take, but something didn't feel right. I wasn't sure how to share this gut feeling, but once I shared with her that it didn't seem to be what she really wanted to do, she immediately burst out crying and admitted that the thought of taking the job was almost unbearable. She later proceeded to build an impressive professional path and landed her dream job.

Choice: Choosing Care and Compassion Above Anything Else

When working with people, we get at times irritated, overwhelmed, scattered, or even bored. Usually when we experience one of these feelings, it means we are either missing something or need to self-manage. There are many actions we can take. One would be to admit at the moment that we are baffled. We can choose to show curiosity. Yet, how you as the coach would seek within yourself is critical, for the most compassionate have the power to allow an energetic shift. Done lovingly, the impact will be significant. In many of these situations, unclear feelings expose the vulnerability of your coachee. It is often a lead worth following. In this case, your care will function as a safety net to foster a new understanding or movement.

Be the Human You Are

It's extremely challenging to lead from your professional persona. You probably have many skills, abilities, and knowledge. Yet, your coachee won't benefit from all of them as much as long as you bring forward a limited and narrow presence of yourself. Being authentic is also an explicit request from your coachee to do the same. Showing your softer and vulnerable sides invites the fullest expression of the both of you. Clearly hearing their unique voice is the ultimate aim of our coachee. This is not an invitation to disclose everything about yourself. It is a calling for your full presence.

Organizational Coaching Sphere: Extending Love Beyond Individuals While

Enhancing Effectiveness in Organizational Coaching

The organizational coaching sphere refers to group coaching activities, such as workshops or training events. Most of the individual coaching practices can also be transcended to the organizational coaching sphere, with a few additions. Encouraging the participants to lovingly notice their peers will multiply the effectiveness of any group coaching, even if the aim isn't team building or another form of ongoing collaboration. The coach supports that by creating initial and ongoing opportunities for the participants to present their best selves and their positive reactions. This action will allow a connection to be formed.

Expressing Gratitude: The Coach as a Role Model

Modeling Love and Gratitude: Demonstrating the Impact of Love

As the leading force of the group, you are the role model. When you are genuinely taking part in the experience and demonstrate your impressions, others will follow. Feeling your excitement and care, the participants will become highly engaged and much more inclined to play along. Their feeling of comfort to be at ease with the group will grow.

From Awareness to Action: Embracing Love as Your Coaching Default Mode

By consistently choosing care and compassion above anything that comes up, you foster an environment where your coachees can explore, learn, and grow. Leading from your fullness and open heart brings an additional value that leading from a limited professional self can't. Being authentic is also an explicit request from your coachee to do the same. Ultimately, love can become your coaching default mode, creating a lasting and transformative impact.

A Loving Legacy: The Ripple Effect of Coaching with Love

Be it in personal coaching relationships or within the organizational coaching sphere, love has the power to create a ripple effect, spreading from the fulfilled hearts of your coachees to their surroundings and onwards. Fortunately, love is a renewable and endless resource, multiplying with each loving expansion.

ACTIVITY

Coachee's Essence—Harnessing the Love

If not directed intentionally, your love might not be as powerful as it can. Create an intentional laser of love to scan your coachee with.

This worksheet is designed to be filled out at the beginning of the work process with a new coachee.

It can also be used when an additional loving reminder is needed during mid-process.

The Search

A coach seeks the most inner truth. One that is not disguised as shields.

Name five essence attributes of your coachee:

1.

2.

3.

4.

5.

The Skillful Offering

Being brave in this context means staying focused on the necessity of the truth.

What are the truths your coachee prefers to look away from? (It is not about having an assumption! It is about feeling the human in front of you and continuing to assess as you go along.)

1.

2.

3.

4.

5.

Meeting With Love

Whether it is holding the space or person with the assumption of love or finding the proper manner to shout the love outwards.

List your intuition—which offerings of love would be most beneficial for your coachee? (It can be a smile, a certain expression while listening, or loving words.)

1.

2.

3.

4.

5.

About the Author

From very early on, Ya'ara Segal found herself fascinated with words, ideas, and the people around her. During her life's journey, she kept uncovering magical layers of literal joy within pages of human stories composed by others and later by her own bubbling mind.

As a life coach and trainer, she holds expertise in supporting people to compose their own accurate life narrative. Ya'ara's current professional focus lies in training and supporting job coaches who are accompanying refugees integrating into the Swiss IT market. Ya'ara is dedicated to transforming the culture of division, and passionately employs coaching as a powerful tool to foster unity and positive change.

Prior to becoming a coach, Ya'ara was a loving literature high school teacher with the biggest number of classes for two years in a row. That means she had to decipher around 200 pages of teenagers' handwriting per exam season.

Ya'ara was born and raised in Israel and has been living in Zurich since 2013. She is sharing accommodation with her funny and wise family members.

Get in touch with Ya'ara at Yaara.bea@gmail.com or follow her work at https://www.linkedin.com/in/ya-ara-segal-cpcc-931234a5/

CHAPTER 20

Uniting Spirituality, Health, and Creative Expression for Personal Growth

By Judy E. Slater
CEO of Innerlude & Associates, Life Coach
Novato, California

Also, go inside and listen to your body because your body will never lie to you. Your mind will play tricks, but the way you feel in your heart, in your guts, is the truth.

—Don Miguel Ruiz

The longest relationship you have is the one with your body. Listen to it! Treat it with love and care, and you will know your truth, and your truth will set you free.

You are a spiritual being living in a human body. You are a perfectly imperfect beloved child of the Divine Benevolent Source of Love. You are loved more than you will ever know. You have been wounded, have wounded others, and have a broken "love bond."

Yet love is a steadfast constant that survives everything, and you must heal yourself so that you can in turn help heal the world. You are created to be creative. You have a unique set of abilities, gifts, skills, talents, and some important piece of truth to offer the world. These beliefs form the foundational triad for my coaching practice and working with clients.

The Core Strand of the Triad Is Spirituality

Spirituality is concerned with the human spirit or soul as opposed to material or physical things. It is the broad concept of a belief you have in something beyond the self. It may or may not be a mental assent to a proposition; it may be a radical trust, loyalty, or allegiance to something or someone, or a way of seeing the world. You believe in something, or you would not be alive.

Spirituality is not a single path or belief system. Your beliefs and spirituality are based on everything you have experienced in life and their created worldview. Your worldview is largely unconscious and includes your assumptions, attitudes, behaviors, beliefs, communication style, genetic makeup, values, the way you process information, everything you experience in your body, your family, your community, your work environment and norms, your culture, your geographic region, and your natural world, which all work together to shape your own unique filter of reality. Your worldview is reflected in your values, which are a key tool used in coaching.

There are many ways to experience spirituality, the benefits of spirituality, and each spiritual experience. It's a great challenge to all of us who live in a busy 21st century world, for practicing spiritual disciplines is never simple. And one of the concepts I use to broaden a client's awareness of their spirituality is through what I call "vital practices" rather than the classic term "spiritual disciplines." I've expanded the typical spiritual disciplines of celebration, confession, fasting, forgiveness, hospitality, meditation, prayer, reconciliation, service, solitude, stewardship, and worship to include others, which may look more "secular" than "sacred." Any intentional activity that turns your awareness more fully to the Divine Benevolent Source of Love is a vital practice, for they are absolutely necessary, important, essential for life, full of energy, and life giving. Don't you like that? Any activity can have a spiritual component and be vital for your own life. The possibilities are endless.

So what do you need to do to feel alive?

For me, it is standing in the presence of great art. For friends of mine, it's hiking, biking, walking, doing yoga, or tai chi. For others, it's journal writing, poetry, painting, sculpture, photography, creating something, cooking, gardening, and even laughing: anything that in its own way makes your heart and whole body sing with vibrant energy. It's something that if you don't do it daily or often, your spirit dies. And it may not be something that you do alone. There are communal practices as well such as sharing a meal, dancing, singing, cheering on a favorite sports team, the list is endless. The clue is when you aren't doing it, you feel deadened, dull, down.

Vital practices change your heart. They form a bridge between being and doing and become living pictures of divine intention for a world of love and justice. They are personal practices, not programs or products. They are not things you do in order to be loved and accepted but are things that are done to you in response to grace because of divine love and the desire for you as a beloved child of the Divine Benevolent Source of Love.

Challenge yourself and your clients to commit to three to five minutes a day of being present with a vital practice. Engage in one personal practice and one communal practice and ask: Where is the divine spirit active here? What kind of person might I become if I consistently devote myself to my chosen vital practices?

The Second Strand of the Triad Is Health

Ninety-nine percent of all illnesses are caused by a broken "love bond," leaving an imprint on the entire system across time. You have been wounded, wounded others, and suffer trauma in some form. In other words, you share not only a family consciousness but a universal consciousness of trauma that is stored in your body and psyche that wants and needs to be healed in order to regain vibrant health and vitality. It must be healed by releasing the stuck, stored energy in the body.

For energy is the foundational basis of all life, linking everything in the universe in an energetic interdependence. Your thoughts are energy and create your reality. Your emotions are energy in motion, and your body uses energy to act as well as store energy. Illness arises when the energy stored is not your own but other people's, which is referred to as other people's energy or OPE. Thus, to heal, you must release any foreign energy with the goal of being 100% full of yourself (yes, pun intended), 100% of the time. One of the practices to do this is called Neutral Separations, which is the activity at the end of the chapter you can use for yourself and for your clients. You must heal yourself so that you can heal the world. And you must focus on the body to heal.

There are three centers of intelligence: the mind, the heart, and the body, and each of them provides you with basic skills you use to make decisions about life. Different situations require primary use of one of them. For example, your mind is the best choice for gathering and analyzing information, figuring out new ways of doing things and making plans. Your heart or emotional center is the best choice to feel your feelings and the messages they point to underneath, be sensitive to emotional reactions, connect with others emotionally, and guide your decisions in relationships. Your body center, or movement center, is the best choice for taking action, getting into motion, experiencing physical sensations, taking control of your environment, and releasing any dis-ease.

As a society, we favor the mind and intellect and use them to express our thoughts, draw conclusions, and make decisions based on facts and reasoning. It is not the best intelligence for healing illness, although learning the behavior, patterns, and thoughts that contributed to illness is helpful. At the same time, we devalue our heart or emotional intelligence by holding back any hint of emotional expression and often apologize for spontaneous emotional expression as something we should not be showing or sharing. And far behind the mind and the heart, the body intelligence is the least acknowledged as an intelligence, for it is instinctual and intuitive, happens almost instantaneously, and then is gone. It is also the least listened to for we have devalued our bodies as animalistic, out of control, objectified, and unreliable.

We must raise the recognition and reliance of our body intelligence not only in everyday life but in our coaching sessions. Pay attention to body language: non-verbal communication based on posture, eye movement, facial expressions, gestures, mannerisms, touch, and the use of space. Pay attention to the physical sensations that arise from your gut area, the intuitive flashes that appear around or just outside your body, and the way your body wants to move spontaneously when a name, subject, or task is offered. Learn how and where your body speaks to you. Let your body speak, listen to what it says, then act on it for your and your client's best health and vitality.

Ask your clients what and where they are noticing or sensing (do not use the word "feeling" as that is related to emotions), the reaction or response to something said or what is in the space. Learn simple non-verbal energy release techniques, find a bodyworker or energy healer to work with, or commit to a movement practice such as belly breathing, dance, exercise, martial arts, qi gong, shaking, stretching, swimming, tai chi, yoga, or walking. Many can be modified to accommodate limitations.

The Third Strand of the Triad Is Creative Expression

Creativity means to add something worthwhile to the world. True creativity is an attitude you bring to life, how you attend to, experience, and value whatever is present for you in the moment. Creativity means being who you are, finding words, images, and expressions for your feelings, sensations, and thoughts. By its very nature, creativity is a deviant act. It brings new things into being, sees things in new and fresh ways, and allows you to translate your inner life into outward forms, as unique and expressive as you are. Everyone has an instinct for creativity, to share something with the world in some way. Creativity is the basis of your survival. It's a matter of life and death. Being made in the image of the Creator means that you are a creator and co-creator with the Divine Benevolent Source of Love. And you are most divinely inspired when you exercise your creative impulses and display your passionate emotions, for these are the bodily energies that manifest in self-expression, stimulate transformation, and provoke global change.

To create is to risk. Fear and distrust keep you from creating and keeps your heart small and sickly. Creativity is an experience that takes the courage and trust to risk and explore the depths of yourself and the world's struggles. Creativity is wild power, energy that happens at the border between chaos and order. It's a combination of making things happen and letting things happen. Thus, to be in the act of creating grows your heart, heals you deeply, and gives you the courage to see the bigger picture of your life and world, so you can grow into that bigger vision and truth of life itself.

This can only happen in a safe environment, one where there is a sense of safety and self-acceptance, safety from criticism and judgment, freedom of expression, respect for uniqueness, and unconditional love. This space is what you as a coach must create and offer in order for your clients to become the courageous creators you know them to be. Offer them a space that allows the faith to relinquish control and give way to joy, mystery, surprise, and surrender, not just to creativity but to living a fulfilled life.

Being creative does not mean being artistic. In fact, I ban the "A" word, for "artist" is a temperament or personality type and is not necessarily based on talent or skills.

Rather, creativity is universal and can be seen in some of the usual places and many you might just gloss over like begetting and nourishing children, care for family and friends, cleaning, collecting, cooking a meal, curiosity, dressing in your own unique style, experimenting, playing games, gardening, home décor and renovation, humor and wit, improv, influencing, leadership, negotiating, nature ecology, problem solving, public speaking, relationships, running a business, self-expression, science projects and research, strategy, tactics, teaching, thinking, toy making, travel, wonder, working with animals, wrapping packages, worldbuilding, Zen doodling, and anything else that shares who you are with the world. The options really are endless. Everyone is creative, active, curious, energetic, free, interesting, interested, and part of a vast creative universe, past, present, and future. And you have a unique set of creative abilities, gifts, skills, talents, and some important piece of truth to offer the world.

Most often, you and your client's thoughts about themselves as a creative being have been blocked by dreams lost as a child when someone close to you or cultural expectations told you that you were not good enough. You were criticized and judged. Humor and teasing were used to demean and diminish you. You were shamed. All of this discouraged you to learn, practice, and engage your curiosity and courage, thus breaking or shattering the "love bond."

Your work as a coach is to help your client restore their innate creative spark and help them find their unique means of expressing themselves. Simple ways of doing this include asking them to choose a color, image, song, or symbol they can use to express the discovery from a coaching session and put it in a place where they can see it often: wallpaper on their phone or computer, card, picture, or token that reminds them of their creativity. These don't require any "artistic abilities" on their part, and yet you can encourage them to add to, embellish, and make it their own in any way they want. Be sure to ask them to share it with you. And ask them how it makes them feel and what they learned from it. Let creative expression be part of their vital practices and healing.

The Three Strands Woven Together Create the Holistic Path to Flourishing

Know who you are, just as you are, as a perfectly imperfect beloved child of the Divine Benevolent Source of Love. Be present in each moment in an energetic state of health and well-being by being 100% full of yourself. And attend to life with creative expression, curiosity, humility, joy, wonder, and perhaps a deviant act or two.

May you and your clients truly flourish in life.

ACTIVITY

Neural Separations

One of the easiest ways to discard other people's energy (OPE) is by practicing Neutral Separations, which distinguishes your life force energy from OPE and empowers your personal energy and boundaries, as well as allowing greater objectivity and self-expression, thus creating a healthier, more harmonious relationship rather than unhealthy merging and draining of energy. Use it after any energy exchange with individuals, or follow the protocol below for group neutral separations for groups of people, organizations, and objects such as computers, etc.

Neutral Separations for an Individual

- Centered in your meditation sanctuary (the intersection of your ears and the top of your head), intuit a person you choose to make energy separations from.
- Greet the person spirit to spirit and hold an image, knowing, symbol, etc., representing the person outside of your aura (the energetic skin outside your body).
- Note five neutral, objective points of difference between you and that person.
- Sense the uniqueness of each of you as individuals.

Neutral Separations for groups, organizations, or objects such as computers:

- Centered in your meditation sanctuary (the intersection of your ears and the top of your head), intuit the group or object and simply place them outside your energy field on a bus, in a space capsule, whatever you imagine and create.

Continue for Both Individuals and Groups, Organizations, or Objects:

- Intentionally release their energy from your space and gift it back to them, using the hand gesture of palms facing out, pushing toward them.
- Intentionally call back your energy from them, using the hand gesture of palms facing and moving towards you.
- Receive your energy and draw it into your life force, receive it back into your body, and ground into present time by using the hand gesture of palms facing the ground.
- Acknowledge ending the communication by being silent for a few seconds.
- Dissolve the image of the person, group, organization, or object, and release thoughts of that person, group, organization, or object.
- Reground in present time again, be in your meditation sanctuary, and fill yourself up with your life force energy.

® Academy of Intuition Medicine, adapted by Judy E. Slater

About the Author

Judy E. Slater is an Edgewalker, drawing from her expertise as an ordained PC(USA) Minister, certified CTI coach and leadership graduate, Intuition Medicine Practitioner ®, trauma wellness educator, and creative expression dilettante. She currently facilitates adaptive leadership cohort groups, offers workshops in building resilience in times of burnout, stress, and trauma, is a TA at the Academy of Intuition Medicine ®, and co-founder of C Street Village Cohousing. She fosters rabbits, quilts, exposes herself to art, nature, and travel, flourishing in life. Her lifetime journey of self-love found the biggest block to feeling loved, accepted, and worthy of love was herself. Out of this yearning for others to experience self-love, *The Simply Self-Wonderful Card Deck* and companion *The Simply Self-Wonderful Inner Workout Book* were blessed into being in late 2023.

Learn more at www.simplyselfwonderful.com and how to work with Judy at www.innerludecoach.com Her email address is innerludecoach@gmail.com

Judy and Innerlude and Associates can also be found on Facebook and LinkedIn.

CHAPTER

21

The Career Fulfillment Accelerator—For Coaching Clients Navigating a Career Change

By Holly Smevog, MS, ACC
Founder, HMS Consulting, Career & Life Coach
Portland, Maine

*When I'm inspired, I get excited because I can't
wait to see what I'll come up with next.*

—Dolly Parton

When an individual chooses life coaching—looking to make improvements in their life—career satisfaction is often part of the equation. That's no surprise: We spend about one-third of our lives working. As a coach, it's helpful to know some fundamentals about career planning. Without becoming an expert, you can learn tools to help your clients navigate the ins and outs of work and set career goals.

You're a Life Coach and Your Client Needs Career Coaching?

Don't panic if you're a more general life coach and your client needs career coaching specifically. If you're good at what you do as a coach, you already have the right tools to help someone with their career in the most important ways: self-discovery, goal setting, action-planning, and accountability. Armed with the tips and tricks in this chapter, you'll have the template for a process that you can adapt as your own. Let's start with a few basics to help establish a solid foundation to assist you in helping clients with career needs.

How Is "Career" Different from "Job?"

The term "career," which is often used interchangeably with "job," is properly defined as an occupation undertaken for a significant period of a person's life that offers opportunities for progress. The definition implies longevity—debatably a thing of the past—and some evolution or upward mobility.

The most important factor in pursuing a career is a sense of purpose. Finding meaningful work takes on a different form for everyone, and it's the crux of the coaching conversation. How can we help clients find out what will give them the satisfaction and fulfillment to make any one "job" a good fit, and with the potential to become a career?

Holly Smevog, MS, ACC

Life & Career Wheel
Understanding How Clients Have Multiple Roles

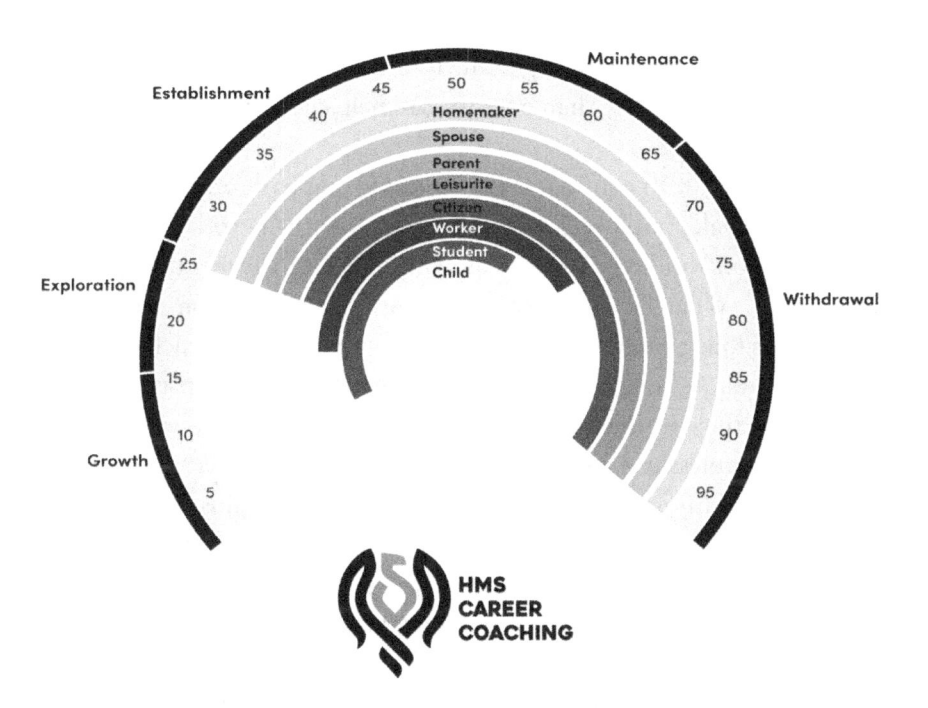

Maintenance
Establishment
Homemaker
Spouse
Parent
Leisurite
Citizen
Worker
Student
Child
Exploration
Withdrawal
Growth

5, 10, 15, 20, 25, 30, 35, 40, 45, 50, 55, 60, 65, 70, 75, 80, 85, 90, 95

HMS CAREER COACHING

A career coach can help a client get perspective on their career depending on their current stage in the life wheel. Explore what roles your client takes on and how that has and may still change based on their age (5-95 represented in the chart).

Current Trends that Impact Career Coaching

It's helpful to be aware of workplace and market trends when coaching clients on their careers. People are living longer. We are approaching the hundred-year life. That means some may want or need to work past age 65 - possibly another ten years. The upside of this reality is that clients have more time to make a career pivot. We see this happening now. The average individual holds 12-plus jobs in a lifetime. The number of times people change careers—apply their skills to a new field of work—is between five and seven. Some clients in their mid-thirties may believe it's too late for a big career change. Much to their surprise, they might find they have time for more than one. We can help clients by normalizing the desire for a change.

Another shift to consider is the increased emphasis on career satisfaction in general. Employees are more critical of their work environment and how work, and relationships at work, impact their mental and physical health. What's more, they are empowered to question the system. Employees today see career satisfaction as something over which they have more control. As coaches, we can encourage clients to assert that control to improve their work environment. And, when needed, to be resilient in the face of professional adversity.

Advances in technology affect employees. On the plus side, new jobs are created every day. However, for clients who are not tech savvy, encountering new technology can be intimidating. Coaching can help reduce the sense of being overwhelmed and introduce practical ways to feel more comfortable with necessary technology. Take artificial intelligence (AI) as an example. AI can be shared with clients as a tool to aid the job search and application process. Cover letters, a highly time-consuming and stressful part of a job search can now be produced much more quickly. As with most things, perspective and a positive outlook can have a huge impact.

The new normal of remote work has introduced positives and negatives. Working parents, single parents, or clients with disabilities may benefit from the flexibility to work from home. On the flip side, remote opportunities are more competitive because they open the door to many more applications. It's also not uncommon to work with clients who have shifted their geographic location—based on the ability to work from anywhere—only to discover that remote work can be isolating and a lot less fulfilling.

Over the past decades, more young adults overall are getting a college degree and entering the workforce with a diploma. Gender roles have shifted since the middle of the 20th century. More women are in the workforce. Competition for white-collar jobs is higher and this changes the job search.

Helping clients prepare for a career shift means we need to be ready to have tough conversations about individual characteristics such as risk tolerance and resilience while simultaneously providing instruction about job-search best practices.

Career Coaching Tactics & The Career Fulfillment Program

The Career Fulfillment Accelerator

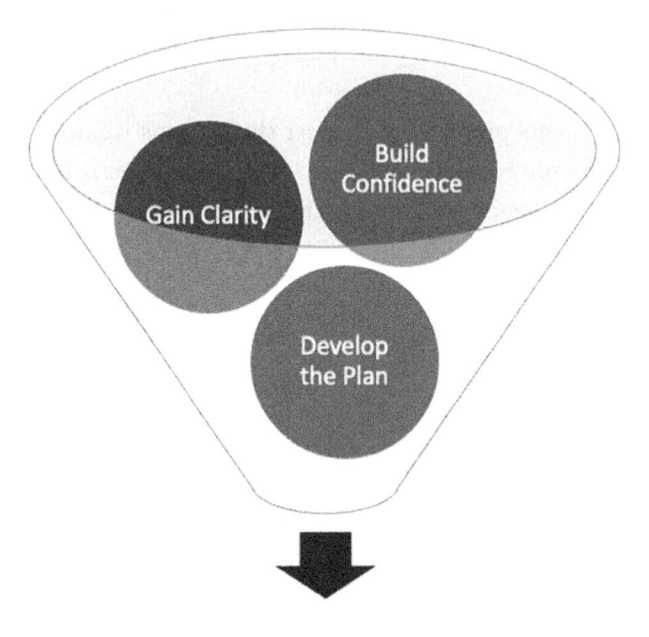

- Gain Clarity
- Build Confidence
- Develop the Plan

⬇

TAKE ACTION & GET RESULTS!

HMB CAREER COACHING

Taking a step-by-step approach to career planning can make a daunting challenge feel achievable. The career fulfillment program—a coaching initiative based on four key pillars—can be applied with success to most career coaching challenges. Beginning with a thorough process of self-discovery and ending with a plan that you, as the coaching partner, help put into action, this program has numerous benefits for clients. The result is often something they never expected. Trust the journey of this process.

Pillar One: Building Confidence with the Strengths and Values Inventory

During the initial session, it's helpful to learn a bit about your client's past with a focus on professional history. How did they get to where they are today? What decisions did they make along the way and what factors went into the decision-making process? What experiences, training, and education are they bringing to the table? It's important to let clients share their sense of self and their world view. Listen and learn. Probe to learn more but save your questions and hypotheses for later.

Assessments offer a wonderful complement to initial coaching sessions. A helpful trio is a values assessment, a personality assessment, and a skills assessment. Free assessments can be found online if you are not licensed to administer more formal instruments. Assessments do not give answers. Their value is to add quantitative information to otherwise qualitative conversations.

A values assessment will help your client to prioritize what's most important to them. What do they absolutely need from their job? A personality assessment will help clients understand their favored work environment, learning styles and how much they value social interaction. Next, a skills assessment is useful in building your client's confidence by helping them articulate what they can do and what they believe the work world needs them to contribute. Confidence motivates action. And action results in hope, which encourages more confidence, more hope, and more action.

Ask your client which skills they would enjoy using every day at work. Skills that are well developed and enjoyable are the most motivating for long-lasting satisfaction in a career. Reflect on the values and skills your client reports and help them pare down the list to a top five for each.

Completed Action: Client feels more confident because they can articulate their top strengths and values.

Pillar Two: Gain Clarity with the Authentic Direction Discovery

Once you have an idea of your client's skills and values, it's time to create a vision by determining where these fit into the world of work. Many career assessments recommend areas of career focus that are particularly helpful for early career planners. The goal for coaching at this stage is to help clients brainstorm ideas for possible careers, industries, and job titles that match their strengths and values. If the list is long, help them carefully weigh the choices against their values—what would life be like if they chose a certain career? Would they have the income, work-life balance, sense of achievement or autonomy they said they really wanted? Drill down to a maximum of three to five choices. Prioritize the first avenues to explore more deeply.

What Dreams Does Your Client Have?

Question for Client: "What's the best-case scenario? A year from now, you wake up and you're excited to go to work and happy with your career. What do you see when you imagine this?" Get the fullest picture you can of what they know about what they want and where the gaps are.

Question for Client: "What could be even better than that?" Clients often get very excited when they think things could be "better than good"; in fact, things could be "great." Generate a little hope in every session.

Collect information about each possible career path. This data can come from multiple sources. For more quantitative information, the Bureau of Labor and Statistics Occupational Outlook Handbook (OOH), Glassdoor, LinkedIn, and other easily accessible online sites provide insights about industry growth outlook, salary standards, educational and training requirements, satisfaction of the population of workers in a certain role, qualifications and more.

In many cases, qualitative information is the ultimate deciding factor. Once clients have a few options in mind, help them find people to talk to—people who are in the role they want, people who hire for the role they want, etc. Some clients will want to volunteer in an organization, take a class in the field, or become part of an industry association as ways to further evaluate their interest and fit in a given path.

Completed Action: Clients are energized with one to three career options, they are collecting data to evaluate the choices, and they're excited to move forward.

Pillar Three: Focus Action with the Career Transition Plan

Crafting an action plan generates excitement and momentum. Clients feel more hopeful and believe they can achieve the career happiness they want. Hope is motivating. Hope supports the resilience and perseverance clients need to navigate their career change. As a coach, it's important to support this mindset so that clients maintain a positive outlook and keep moving forward. One way is to develop a plan with logical milestones that are easily achievable and still rewarding.

For career changers, the biggest steps in an action plan will be developing a list of target employers, identifying best fit opportunities, and making connections with people, otherwise known as networking.

The first part—finding opportunities and employers—is often based on your client's chosen field of work. Other variables can be geography, reputation, mission, and connections. This aspect of the job search is more research-based and easier for the client to pursue on their own.

Often the coaching needs to focus on networking. A career coach helps clients realize the breadth of their possible connections, feel confident enough to reach out to people, and understand how to approach the communication. It's worth assessing how the message lands and to make sure the client isn't overwhelming or off-putting.

Help your client set weekly goals and encourage them to maintain progress. For instance, a typical full-time job seeker could make seven to ten connections per week. In any networking conversation, clients should be reminded to be more curious about the other person and wait to talk about themselves when asked. People are more likely to help others when they feel heard and appreciated.

Clients may need help preparing for a networking appointment. They should have a professional statement or elevator pitch per the example below. The person they're speaking to should easily understand what they do or what they seek. Clients should be ready to answer the question "How can I help you?" and make it easy for the contact to provide that help.

Elevator Pitch Template: *I am a [industry professional] with deep experience in [area of expertise]. My strengths include [strength #1] and [strength #2]. I have achieved [accomplishment #1] and [accomplishment #2], and I am interested in building [career goal] in my next role.*

Remind clients to ask for new people to contact as a part of each networking conversation. For example, "Who else do you think I should be reaching out to?" They are likely to get one, two or three names; this is how to build significant momentum in this most challenging phase of the job search.

The networking process has several goals. Clients must "get the word out" that they are looking for a job and elicit help when it's appropriate and offered. They should collect information to inform themselves about what they would like to do and for whom, and build relationships in the context of their potential career.

Completed Action: Client feels enough certainty about next steps to have networking conversations and has a plan in place that ensures timely progress.

Pillar Four: Build Momentum with the Career Builder's Toolkit & Coaching Accountability

By this time, your client feels confident, has clarity about next steps, is making connections, is getting validation and support from others, and is ready to move into full action mode. As a coach, you can help your client enter the job market with the right messaging and professional branding. This includes a resume, cover letter, LinkedIn profile, and any other media or materials required. There are many freelance consultants who can assist if helping with these materials is not in your sphere. Your client needs to be talking about themselves in ways that their audience, such as hiring managers, recruiters, and networking contacts, understand.

Branding tip: The top of the resume and the top of the LinkedIn profile are the most important fields on these pages. The key words next to your name make an instant impression on the reader. Make sure your client references the exact keywords used in job postings.

Your role as a coach includes helping your client create a positive vision for their future career. From there, the coach guides the client through a process of self-discovery that results in confidence and hope. Hold your client accountable to the action plan, recognize and celebrate wins, help your client over bumps in the road, and encourage resilience.

The average job search or career pivot takes up to six months. During that time, almost everyone will make mistakes, encounter rejection, and feel discouraged. That is all normal.

Deploy coaching skills to inspire, motivate, and energize clients. Most people do not see how great they are. They downplay their skills and achievements. Occasionally, plans get adapted or revised along the way, but most often, commitment to the goal and an optimistic outlook gets results.

Completed Action: Client takes ownership over career transition, feels supported in the journey and starts to see results!

ACTIVITY

Authentic Direction Discovery Worksheet

Strengths
Skills I would be happy using every day.

1.
2.
3.
4.
5.

Values
The most important things I need and want from work.

1.
2.
3.
4.
5.

Roles to Explore
Where my skills and values come together in the world of work?

1.
2.
3.
4.
5.

What actions will I take now to find information about these roles?

1.
2.
3.
4.
5.

What questions do I need answered to make the right choice?

1.
2.
3.
4.
5.

HMS CAREER COACHING

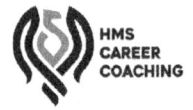

About the Author

Holly Smevog, ACC, CCC, founded HMS Career Coaching in 2018. Holly has a professional mission of connecting people with their best career. She is a globally certified career counselor through the National Career Development Association (NCDA) and International Coaching Federation Associate Certified Coach (ICF ACC), experienced and approved to apply counseling, coaching, and consulting skills to each client engagement. From Silicon Valley to Southern Maine, Holly's diverse background includes marketing and product development, consumer product design and sales, instructional technology and training, and human resource consulting. With experience in both the public and private sectors and in organizations large and small, Holly has an in-depth understanding of what makes companies succeed and how people work best together. She has helped hundreds of individuals overcome career obstacles and find their vocational sweet spot.

Email: holly@hmscareercoaching.com
Website: https://hmscareercoaching.com/
Instagram: https://www.instagram.com/hmscareercoaching/
LinkedIn: https://www.linkedin.com/in/hollysmevog/

CHAPTER 22

Curiosity Didn't Kill the Cat, and It Won't Kill You

By Ryan Spence
Integrative Life Coach, Author of *The Triple C Method*®
Sheffield, England, United Kingdom

Live a life full of humility, gratitude, intellectual curiosity, and never stop learning.

—GZA

What makes a good coach?

Actually, let's aim higher than that: What makes a great coach? It's a question that focuses the mind, encouraging you to reflect on the work you're doing and how you're doing it. It's the question that often comes up in communities of coaches, provoking spirited and thoughtful debate.

Common answers I've heard include:

- "A great coach is someone who can hold space for clients."
- "A great coach is someone who actively listens without judgment."

- "A great coach is someone who sees more for their client than they see for themselves."

All great responses to a big question. And although it's all subjective, in reflecting on my work as a coach, my clients, and my experience as a coaching client, I believe I've found the answer.

Okay, maybe not the answer, but my answer. And it's an answer I believe is worth sharing.

But before I do, it's helpful for you to know where I'm coming from and how my experiences have shaped what I share with you in this chapter.

I'm an integrative life coach. This means I integrate a number of ideas, beliefs, and modalities into my coaching, including yoga, breath work, and hypnosis, but everything stems from a solid foundation. Just as a tree begins life by planting its roots in the earth, then rises up from the ground by way of its trunk, and from that trunk a myriad of branches emerge, I've found that the work of the best coaches is underpinned by solid roots.

My roots, the foundation of the work I do with my clients, is my coaching framework, the Triple C Method.

The Triple C Method originated during a period of soul searching, which ultimately led me to walk away from an 11-year career as an international finance lawyer at a top ten law firm, a BigLaw lawyer, and take a leap into the unknown as a self-proclaimed BigLaw dropout.

To paraphrase Netflix co-founder Reid Hoffman, I jumped off a cliff, a successful career cliff, and tried to figure out how to build an airplane on the way down.

I'm still trying.

The Triple C Method

But what helped me to get to the point where I could take that leap without knowing how or where I would land are the 3 Cs that form the Triple C Method: clarity, confidence, courage.

And those 3 Cs are a bedrock that have served me and my clients well in creating a life we want rather than settling for a life we think we should want.

These 3 Cs are the roots from which success can grow.

I don't mean the success we're conditioned to chase after: money, status, and a corner office in a gleaming tower of glass and steel. I mean success as you define it, success on your terms.

But what I've realised in my work as a coach and through constant reflection on the question that opened this chapter is that what's missing from the Triple C Method is a fourth C. Staying with the visual image of the tree, if the 3 Cs are the roots, then this fourth C is the trunk. The spine of every coaching conversation.

Now, this C sounds obvious. It sounds like the simplest thing you can do as a coach. But when—

- You're an enthusiastic coach.
- You can see the path you think your client should take or the decision they should make.
- You desperately want to lovingly push your client in what you think is the right direction.

Then it can be easy to forget this C. See, as coaches, we want to help our clients. It's why we do the work we do. We want to help them avoid the pain we see ahead for them and steer them toward less choppy waters. But tempting as that may be, that's not our job. We're the co-passenger, not the driver. And by keeping this fourth C in mind, we can ensure we remain firmly in the passenger seat as our client's helpful guide rather than take their place in the driver's seat of their life.

So what is this mystery C?

Curiosity.

Now, curiosity gets a bad rap sometimes. We're conditioned to dismiss curiosity and instead follow in the footsteps of those who went before us, regardless of whether those footsteps lead to where we want to go.

I mean, I'm sure as an inquisitive child, asking a few too many questions of your parents or a teacher, you heard the common phrase, "Curiosity killed the cat," as a way to shut you down and stop you from seeking answers. You probably heard it so many times that eventually you just stopped asking.

Curiosity Didn't Kill the Cat, and It Won't Kill You

But here's the thing. In using this to dampen your enthusiasm, intrigue, and curiosity, the purveyors of this phrase ignored its evolution, an evolution that reframes its meaning. In the early 1900s in a newspaper in the US, a second part was added to this much used phrase: "Curiosity killed the cat, but satisfaction brought it back." Those additional five words place a whole new spin on it now, right? Instead of curiosity leading to your (or the cat's) doom, it opens you up to opportunities that deliver satisfaction and bring you back to life. A resurrection if you wish.

But this isn't a chapter about the intricacies of 100-plus-year-old phrases. This is a chapter about coaching. Yet I share this because if I had to choose one quality above all others, a quality that with intentional practice can turn a good coach to a great coach, it would be curiosity.

Why?

Because, for the reason previously stated, we're so conditioned to bury our curiosity, follow the well-trodden path to prescribed success, and show up as the expert with all the answers. You see it in the scripts set forth in many a coaching book or seminar. If you dogmatically lead your client through your prescribed process or script, make assumptions about their situation that accord with your life blueprint, and lead them to where you believe they should go, you make your client dependent on you for their growth and success, when the very nature of coaching is to empower your client to recognize, find, and trust their own knowing.

And, perhaps worse than that, over the long term, the client will end up dissatisfied with you, their progress, and themselves because they never got to the essence of what they really wanted and why they really wanted it because you, the coach, thought you knew best and projected your ideas upon them.

See, we're all conditioned to think a certain way, act a certain way, and be a certain way, and if we don't maintain self-awareness of this and intentionally detach from the outcome, we do a disservice to our clients.

Our clients are best served when we approach sessions as an enquiry exercise. When we listen to a client's words and watch their actions from a place of genuine curiosity. When we seek the answers and meaning from them, rather than projecting our own answers and meaning upon them.

I didn't always think this way though.

Beaten down by years in BigLaw, I felt a sense of levity when I finally made the leap out of that world. Through my own personal development quest and coaching journey, I'd managed to break out of the mental cell of self-limitation that had led me to believe I could never be anything other than a BigLaw lawyer, and step through my portal of possibility to enter a world of limitless opportunity.

I felt joyful and excited at the prospect of designing my life instead of living it the way I thought I should. I felt I'd suddenly been handed a secret code or key to the door of my aforementioned mental cell, and I wanted to share it with everyone, so they could stop languishing in lethargy and start living life lit!

And fuelled by my frustration, anger, and injustice at the reality of BigLaw life failing to live up to the dream, like a firefighter whose mission is to rescue people from the burning building, my mission was to rescue everyone in my position—all the unhappy, unfulfilled lawyers I'd met along the way—from the law.

But in the early stages of setting out on that mission, I realised that if I saw every client as needing rescuing and coached them with this pre-determined aim, I'd be projecting my desires and experiences onto them. And when I dug down further into why I wanted to be a coach, it wasn't to lead people down my path, but to guide them back to their own inner knowing, so they could carve their own path and find themself.

That was my light-bulb moment. That was when I resolved to ensure I met each client with curiosity.

But curiosity for curiosity's sake isn't in the best service of your client. Anyone can ask random questions; that's just being nosey. Curiosity isn't just about asking questions; it's being intentional about the questions you ask.

Why are you asking that?

Where are you trying to get the client to go?

What are you trying to get the client to learn about themselves?

Sounds good in the abstract, right? But you're probably thinking, "How does it play out in practice?"

I'm glad you asked.

My client, Jane (not her real name) thought she had a time problem. She felt she was always chasing her tail and never had enough time in a

Curiosity Didn't Kill the Cat, and It Won't Kill You

day to do anything for herself. A high-flying executive, wife, and mum of two, Jane felt she spent all of her time catering to other people's needs, often at the expense of her own. Now, approaching this issue as someone who's felt the same way before, I could have assumed I knew exactly what the problem was and immediately launched into suggesting various time management techniques that Jane should try to create more time for herself, like block time, the Pomodoro Technique, or waking up at 5 a.m. and establishing a morning routine.

But putting on my curiosity cap, I knew that wouldn't be helpful for two reasons.

1. If you've ever shared a problem with someone and had them fire back generic "solutions," you'll know that despite the best intentions, it can make you feel unheard and unsupported.
2. There was so much I didn't know about her situation.

I didn't know if Jane had already tried any of those techniques. I didn't know the source of her problem: Was it a lack of awareness of time management tools, or was something else at play here?

Without that information, me throwing around suggestions like an untethered water hose, however well meaning, would have made the coaching session about me and my solution to the perceived problem, instead of making it about Jane and her actual problem.

So I didn't do any of that.

Instead, I listened actively as she shared her frustrations. And when she stopped, I got curious and asked my first question.

"Why? Why do you think you don't have enough time?"

In a tone that screamed, "Isn't it obvious?" she replied, "Because I'm busy."

"Busy doing what?" I asked, fully aware that given the tone of her response to my previous question, this question was likely to further irritate her. The conversation continued.

"What do you mean—'busy doing what?' Have you been listening to me?"

Her irritation level was rising now. Where it started at maybe a 3, it was now around a 6 and threatening to rise further. But I persisted.

"Yes, I've been listening. And I appreciate all the hats you feel you have to wear. But I'm curious about whether you really have to wear them. So indulge me, take me through your day yesterday, what did you do?"

Annoyed, but seeing that I wasn't letting this go, Jane began to run through the events of her previous day. She raced through it at first, only delivering the headlines.

"I went to work, had a busy day of meetings, went home, had dinner with the family, watched some TV, went to bed."

But maintaining my curiosity and risking a level ten irritation blowout, I continued pressing for more detail with questions like:

"What time did you wake up?"
"What time did you get out of bed?"
"What did you do before you went to work?"
"How long were you in meetings at work?"
"Why did you have to be present at those meetings?"
"What time did you leave the office?"
"How did you get home?"
"What did you do as soon as you stepped in the door at home?"
"Did you make dinner or was it made for you?"
"What time did you eat dinner?"
"What did you do immediately after dinner?"
"What did you watch on TV?"
"How long did you watch?"
"Were you doing anything else while you watched?"

Question, after question, after question. But each question was intentional. Each question had a purpose.

I was curious about how Jane spent her time, and I wanted her to get curious too. And at some point during me playing the part of that inquisitive child we all have hidden away inside of us, her irritation level started to drop as a metaphorical light bulb appeared above her head.

And at that point, I knew a mindset shift had occurred. She was now getting curious too. As the session progressed, sometimes she'd repeat my question back to me, the cogs of her mind whirring as she pondered it.

"Hmmm, what was the purpose of my presence at that meeting?"
"Where did the couple of hours after putting the kids to bed go?"
"Why did I feel the need to log in and check my emails after dinner?"

Like a game of tennis, I'd serve up a question, she'd return an answer, and my curiosity would bat another question right back at her until we got to the root of the problem of where her time was going and whether she had to continue spending it the way she did.

She realised she didn't.

By allowing her curiosity to guide her deeper into the stories she'd been telling herself, she realised that many of the demands she felt were being placed on her by others, she was actually placing on herself.

She didn't need to be at every meeting she was invited to.

She didn't have to prepare and cook every meal for her family.

She didn't have to take her laptop home every night and check emails while she watched TV.

By getting curious, she discovered that it wasn't a question of needing to create more time. It wasn't a question of implementing productivity or time management techniques. It was a question of intentionally spending the time she already had. She thought she had to do certain things, so she did them. And people expected her to do certain things because she had always done them. They had become habitual to the point where much of her day was spent on autopilot, never questioning whether what she was about to do was the way she needed or wanted to spend her time.

As I said before, it would have been easy for me to have opened the session by accepting her story that she had no time and bombarding her with tools and techniques. But without figuring out whether those tools and techniques were appropriate for her specific situation, she would have left the session dissatisfied and never implemented the techniques.

So, my friend, get curious.

Curiosity is the key to unlocking your client's mental cell of self-limitation.

Ask purposeful questions that lead your client to what the problem is, not what they, or you, think the problem might be.

And if you're reading this, thinking, "How do I get started? How do I ask questions that guide rather than confuse?" here are four questions to get you started:

1. Why do you feel or believe that?
2. Where's the evidence to support the story you're telling yourself?

3. If you could change one thing about this situation, what would it be?
4. What's the smallest step you could take right now to make that change?

Imagine your curiosity as a spade. With each question, you're digging deeper until you reach your client's inner wisdom. And that inner wisdom is fertile ground from which your client can begin to grow.

The more curious we are about our clients, the more we encourage our clients to be curious about themselves. And in that curiosity, we empower them to sit in the driver's seat of their own life, take the wheel, and cruise to their chosen destination.

ACTIVITY

The Triple C Method

See the Triple C Method as shown in this chapter and get curious.

About the Author

Ryan Spence is a life coach, yoga and meditation guide, and author of the corporate coaching guide, The Triple C Method®.

A first-class law graduate of the University of London, Ryan's prestigious 11-year career in BigLaw involved him in deals that won the Finance Deal of the Year at the 2018 Asia Legal Awards and the 2019 UN Global Impact Award.

When Ryan realised that each rung of the corporate ladder he reached was taking him further from where he wanted to be, he took a leap of faith and set off on a quest to find himself. Driven by his own experience of corporate life, Ryan has become a passionate leader in the corporate well-being and mindset sphere, coaching professionals to find their version of fulfilment, meaning, and joy, so they can move from survival mode to thrival mode.

Ryan lives with his wife and two children in Sheffield, UK.

Website: https://www.iamryanspence.com/
Instagram: @iam_ryanspence
LinkedIn: https://www.linkedin.com/in/ryan-spence-lawyer-coach-corporate-coach/

CHAPTER 23

The 2/10 Rule of Effective Communication

By Jake Stahl
Founder & CEO of Jake Stahl Consulting
Norwich, Connecticut

*The single biggest problem in communication
is the illusion that it has taken place.*

—George Bernard Shaw

Coaching effective communication requires a foundational understanding, not just a superficial knowledge. This is where the 2/10 rule is unique. To truly impart its value to your clients, you must first embody its principles yourself. By learning it, living it, and modeling it, you're not only mastering a technique but paving the way for transformative change in those you coach. Only when you experience the elevated level of communication the 2/10 rule offers, can you genuinely teach its merits.

Now, let's set the scene: Many of your clients, whether they're in sales, leadership roles, or even in their personal lives, often face the challenge of maintaining engaging and productive conversations. They might share with you experiences of feeling unheard, overwhelmed, or unable to steer a conversation effectively. How can you, as their coach, guide them past these hurdles? Enter the 2/10 rule. This is a solution to these challenges, and your pivotal role is to help them internalize and apply it.

The essence of the 2/10 Rule is simple yet impactful: For every two minutes of conversation, there should be an interaction. Then, at the 10-minute mark, the dialogue should open up for questions or reflections. This rhythmic structure ensures that interactions are interspersed at the second, fourth, sixth, and eighth minutes, with a more in-depth engagement at the tenth minute.

The 2/10 rule isn't merely about setting intervals for interaction. Its inception was aimed at crafting the "perfect conversation." While perfection in communication might seem a lofty goal, through decades of experience and refinement, this technique comes strikingly close. What it doesn't claim to do is dictate the content of your discussions. Instead, it emphasizes the cadence, offering guidance on potential content touchpoints. The ultimate goal is not just about facilitating interaction but ensuring that those interactions are rich, meaningful, and mutual.

Now that we've laid the groundwork, let's delve deeper into the mechanics of the 2/10 rule. Understanding its intricacies will be crucial to integrating it into your coaching sessions and ensuring your clients reap its full benefits. Here's how to break it down for your client:

2-Minute Principle:

- Essence: Periodic, meaningful interaction every two minutes.
- Implementation:
    - Open-Ended Questions: "Does that resonate with you?"
    - Feedback Seeking: "Are you following?"
    - Shared Reflections: "Ever encountered something similar?"

This two-minute rhythm does more than break the monotony. It involves the listener actively, ensuring they're more engaged, and the conversation is collaborative.

10-Minute Principle:

- Essence: A deeper dive every ten minutes for reflection and feedback
- Implementation:
    - Topic Summaries: "I've shared a lot. Thoughts?"
    - Open Floor: "Any questions or points of clarity needed?"

This 10-minute pause is a vital cog in understanding. It offers the listener a chance to process, ask, and truly collaborate in the conversation's direction.

Now, as a coach, it's essential to provide your clients with a holistic view of how this tool can be integrated across various communication scenarios. From boardrooms to living rooms, let's explore where the 2/10 rule can be seamlessly woven into the fabric of daily interactions.

Business Presentations

Employees zoning out is common during lengthy presentations. By adopting the 2/10 rule, presenters can retain attention, ensure understanding, and get invaluable feedback in real-time.

Sales Engagements

In a sale, the client's engagement is the dealmaker or breaker. The 2/10 rule shifts a pitch from a mere presentation to a conversation, fostering trust and rapport.

Training Sessions

My training sessions underwent a transformation with the 2/10 rule. Regular check-ins kept participants engaged, turning sessions into interactive, enlightening experiences.

Family Conversations

Even on a personal front, the rule works wonders. Whether it's discussing college options with your teenager or planning a vacation with a partner, the 2/10 rule ensures everyone's involved, valued, and heard.

> *The greatest problem with communication is we don't listen to understand. We listen to reply.*
> —Roy T. Bennett

The 2/10 rule isn't just a conversational guide; it taps into deep psychological needs and principles of effective communication. Here's a list of benefits for your client:

1. Breaking the Monologue: Conversations should be dynamic, a back-and-forth that ensures both parties are engaged. This principle ensures that conversations remain collaborative rather than one-sided. By regularly injecting interactive moments, you ensure that everyone is on the same wavelength. It fosters a sense of inclusivity, ensuring that the listener feels valued and involved, making it less about disseminating information and more about shared understanding.

2. Facilitating Clarity: Misunderstandings can derail any conversation, and the 2/10 rule works as a preventive measure. By checking in every two minutes, you provide an opportunity to address any misconceptions immediately. This periodic checkpoint confirms mutual understanding, ensuring that the conversation progresses based on clarity rather than assumption.

3. Gathering Thoughts: Speaking isn't just about output; it's about strategy. These regular pauses offer the speaker a moment to breathe, collect their thoughts, and adjust their trajectory based on the listener's feedback. It ensures that what follows is coherent, crisp, and attuned to the listener's needs and responses.

4. Maintaining Focus: The human mind isn't designed for prolonged, passive absorption. It thrives on interaction. By setting a predictable rhythm, you anchor the listener's attention. They aren't merely waiting for the talk to end but actively preparing for the next checkpoint, enhancing their attentiveness and retention.

5. Assimilation and Retention: Information delivered in a steady, segmented flow is easier to process. The mind can compartmentalize and assimilate information more efficiently when it's delivered in chunks. The 2/10 rule inherently structures information into manageable pieces, promoting better comprehension and memory retention.

6. Setting Future Conversation Tones: Communication isn't just about the present moment. Every interaction sets a precedent. Regularly practicing the 2/10 rule communicates respect, attentiveness, and value for mutual interaction. Over time, this conditions both the speaker and the listener to anticipate and appreciate these interactive sessions, molding future conversations to be more balanced and engaging.

Coaches, as you introduce your clients to the intricacies of the 2/10 rule, its beauty will soon become evident. It's not unveiling some revolutionary concept but rather refining an instinctual rhythm we've all tapped into during our most engaging conversations. To illuminate its essence, ask your clients to think back on that heartfelt conversation they recall fondly or that business pitch that seemed to naturally flow. The difference between these instances and others? Genuine interaction taking center stage.

Now, the occasional question might arise: "Do we watch the clock all the time?" Clear this up quickly. Highlight that the "2" and "10" are just guidelines, akin to the lane lines on a highway—helping you steer, but not strictly binding. They're building a conversation rhythm, not religiously tracking seconds. Encourage them to pepper in timely remarks, such as "Catching my drift?" or "Does that ring a bell?" climaxing in richer reflections around the 10-minute juncture. The aim? Craft a flowing dialogue, keeping both parties synchronized. And while we label it the "2/10 rule," it's essential for clients to understand that this could just as easily be the "30-second/5-minute rule." The exact timing isn't the core here; it's the consistent cadence of interaction that truly matters.

Let me share a bit about the rule's proven impact. Drawing from my decade of advocating this principle across 47 states and six countries, I've seen its transformative might. From boardrooms to coffee chats, its power to elevate discourse is undeniable. I've seen businesses, when guided by this rule, witness phenomenal revenue boosts, some even doubling or tripling their figures. But don't just fixate on these high-flying corporate milestones. There are countless tales of enhanced customer service interactions, more profound personal ties, and the undeniable connections woven into everyday conversations.

> *Excellent communication doesn't just happen naturally. It is a product of process, skill, climate, relationship and hard work.*
> —Pat McMillan

However, brace your clients for the journey ahead. Mastery of the 2/10 rule isn't instantaneous. They'll grapple with unlearning some long-standing conversational habits. Help them visualize those monologues they've endured, the pitches that felt eternal, and, of course, those moments with "that person" in their life. Adopting the 2/10 rule is less about tweaking a communication style and more about embracing a holistic shift.

Conclude with a dose of encouragement. The route to mastering the 2/10 rule is laden with countless daily interactions, each a golden opportunity. The rhythm might appear challenging initially, but the success formula remains unchanged: keen listening infused with a hearty serving of genuine empathy.

Admittedly, the art of engagement every two minutes can feel a tad unfamiliar at first. So, if your clients find themselves grasping for ways to engage in a conversation, recommend that they echo the sentiment back. This approach works whether they're playing the role of the listener or the speaker. Let's delve into a few examples:

In a Personal Setting:

Friend: "After years of frustration, I finally snapped and quit my job on the spot."
Me: "Seriously? You walked out just like that?"

In a Business Setting:

Colleague: "Given the revenue slide, we might need to reconsider some of our staples."
Me: "You're saying the revenue drop is that significant?"

It's paramount to stress to your clients the transformative nature of this method—it's about fostering genuine, two-sided engagement. By echoing a sentiment or posing a reflective question, they ensure active participation and signal to their conversational partner that they're truly being acknowledged. The subsequent effect? The conversation deepens, paving the way for richer insights.

Now, if your client is on the speaking end, introducing little checkpoints can also be a transformative touch:

In a Personal Setting:

Me: "I've been rambling about my sudden job exit. What's your take on this whirlwind decision?"
Friend: "Honestly? I think it was high time. You've endured enough there."

In a Business Setting:

Me: "I've walked you through the revenue dips and the consequent shifts we're considering. Do the shifts make sense to you?"
Colleague: "Yes, I don't like it, but I get it."

Let's tackle that all-important 10-minute checkpoint. Think of it as a rest stop during a cross-country drive. You've been cruising along, and then you take a breather, admire the view, and ensure both parties are still enjoying the ride together. To illustrate, if your client is the listener:

Friend: "So after a decade, I just walked out of there, deciding I'd had enough."
Me: "Hang on, so after all those years, you just dropped everything and walked out? Have you skipped any juicy bits? I'm all ears!"

In a Business Setting:

Colleague: "The revenue's been taking hits due to several factors we've discussed."
Me: "So, connecting the dots, the past year's sales trajectory has been affected by the variables you mentioned. Is there any nuanced detail I might've missed?"

And if Your Client is the Speaker? Here Are Some Examples:

Me: "I've been relentless, detailing my dramatic job exit saga. What's your perspective on everything I've told you?"
Friend: "I reckon you took a bold step. How do you feel now?"

From the Boardroom:

Me: "I've outlined the revenue challenges. Before I go any further do you have any questions?"
Colleague: "No, I think I'm clear."

The brilliance of the 2/10 rule isn't solely in its structural precision but its chameleon-like adaptability. Whether you're catching up over coffee or presenting in a corporate setting, it molds seamlessly into the conversation.

Now, onto something even more captivating. What if I told you that people value sharing their stories or expertise so much that they'd gladly part with their hard-earned cash just for an attentive audience? Sounds surreal, but it's backed by solid research. Sharing personal stories or insights lights up the same pleasure centers in our brains as landing a $50 bonus or savoring that delicious slice of chocolate cake. We're talking about a neural party, with feel-good vibes all around.

But here's the twist. The human brain, with all its intricate majesty, has this endearing habit: When it consistently feels good around someone, it attributes that warmth to them. It's a form of positive association. So when you lace your conversations with the 2/10 rule, you're not only ensuring effective communication, but you're also enhancing your likability quotient. It's no surprise, then, that individuals who've incorporated this technique have seen improvements ranging from spiking sales numbers, heightened satisfaction scores, to even deeper personal connections.

> *If you just communicate, you can get by. But if you communicate skillfully, you can work miracles.*
> —Jim Rohn

Coaches, when guiding your clients through the art of meaningful communication, it's essential to dissect the nuances of the 2/10 rule, ensuring they understand not just the "how" but the "why."

Begin by clarifying potential misconceptions. Your clients might pose the question, "Aren't the two-minute interactions and the ten-minute reflections pretty much the same thing?" At a cursory glance, they may seem similar. But here's how you can help them discern the distinct intentions.

Introduce the two-minute touchpoints as conversational sparklers. Explain that these brief interludes serve as alert signals, constantly reigniting your client's audience's attention, pulling them back from potential daydreams or mental check-outs. Whether your client is the main speaker seeking affirmation or playing a more passive role, these touchpoints are essential to ensure the conversation's heartbeat remains steady and vibrant.

On the other hand, position the ten-minute marker as a conversational anchor point. It's more than just a pause; it's a profound moment of reflection. Encourage your clients to view this as an opportunity to let their listeners marinate in the conversation's essence. This moment isn't just about a quick check-in; it's about fostering deeper comprehension and ensuring mutual understanding.

While the intentions may seem nuanced, the underlying objectives of these interactions differ profoundly. Use an analogy—liken the two-minute interactions to the fleeting brilliance of a shooting star, and the ten-minute pause to the enduring glow of the moon. Both illuminate the night but in remarkably distinct ways.

Remind your clients that in the symphony of communication, notes of authentic engagement and profound comprehension compose the most memorable melodies. The 2/10 rule is their sheet music, guiding them to craft conversations that transcend mundane chatter. By embedding this rhythm, they'll not just engage; they'll resonate, striking chords often untouched by traditional communication techniques.

Lastly, challenge them. Encourage your clients to integrate the 2/10 rule in their ensuing conversations, whether they're negotiating a business deal, reconnecting with an old friend, or presenting to a team. Urge them to observe the palpable depth it introduces, the strengthened connections it fosters, and the unparalleled clarity it manifests. Let them know: It's about orchestrating conversations that don't merely bounce off the ears but deeply resonate within. Most importantly, it will start you and your client's quest for the perfect conversation.

ACTIVITY

Performing and Coaching "The Perfect Conversation" with the 2/10 Rule

As the coach, do this in every conversation:

1. **Set a timer.** Start by setting a timer for yourself.
2. **Engage every two minutes.** Throughout the conversation, aim to create an interaction every two minutes. Here are a couple of techniques at your disposal:
    a. *Mirroring empathetic statement*
        i. Example:
            1. **Client:** "I'm having trouble sleeping."
            2. **You:** "So sleeping is one of your primary concerns?"
    b. *Asking a Question*
        i. Example:
            1. **Client:** "I'm having trouble sleeping."
            2. **You:** "Do you have trouble getting to sleep or staying asleep?"

3. **Pause and summarize at ten minutes.** Every ten minutes, pause the conversation and perform a brief wrap-up or open it for questions.
    a. Example:
        i. **You:** "We've been talking for a while. Let me summarize where we are, and you can tell me if I missed anything."

The 2/10 Rule of Effective Communication

   ii. **Or:** "We've just covered quite a bit of ground. Do you have any questions about what we've covered over the last ten minutes?"

To allow your client to become proficient, have them repeat this exercise until they gain fluency:

1. **Prepare a ten-minute presentation.** Have your client prepare a ten-minute presentation on any topic of their choice. It can be related to something they are passionate about, a practice business presentation, or simply a discussion of their thoughts and feelings.
2. **Practice the 2/10 Rule.** Instruct them to deliver the presentation to you while practicing the 2/10 Rule.
3. **Create interactions.** They must actively create an interaction with you every two minutes during their presentation.
4. **Open for questions at ten minutes.** At the ten-minute mark, encourage them to open the floor for questions.

Important Note

Remind your clients that this communication method differs from what they've learned previously but has the potential to revolutionize their relationships and enhance their business presentations. Emphasize that mastery takes time and practice, and reassure them that initial struggles are entirely normal—sometimes it might take more than a few attempts. The communication habits they've developed over the years are deeply ingrained, and creating real change will require time and effort. However, the rewards are substantial. They can anticipate deeper and more meaningful conversations, improved relationships through intimate communication, and increased confidence in public speaking or presenting to groups as they gain control over their interactions.

About the Author

Jake Stahl is a pioneer in conversational dynamics and a highly regarded Fractional Chief Learning Officer. He is revolutionizing sales through his "Adaptive Conversational Blueprint," turning sales professionals into relational architects capable of forging profound connections with prospects. Integral to his approach is the 2/10 Rule, which challenges traditional perspectives on conversation and emphasizes the importance of rhythm and cadence. With a rich background spanning 30 years, Jake has shared his expertise in training and development across six countries, impacting over 10,000 individuals. A doting husband and father of four, Jake seamlessly blends practical experience and insightful wisdom in his pursuit of the perfect conversation and empowers businesses through masterful conversations.

Message from the author: If you're reading this book, you're unique. One of the few elite-level people who want to communicate on a level far above everyone else. Reach out to me here to start your journey toward having deeper connections with everyone you meet:

Website: www.jakestahlconsulting.com
LinkedIn: www.linkedin.com/in/jakestahl

CHAPTER 24

The Power to Tap into Your Authentic Self

By Julie Stévigny
Holistic Life Coach, Author of *Love You Latte, Sophie*
Lievegem, Belgium

*Give yourself permission to be every bit of
the woman you are destined to be.*

—UNKNOWN

Isn't it strange that at a young age, let's say five to six years old, you don't need the permission for being yourself, for expressing who you are. You're just you and people (most of them) are okay with that. But once you're an adult, you seek validation for being yourself. You look for permission from others. You hide who you are out of fear, rejection, or disappointment.

As a child, you discover the world just as it is. You see it with your newborn eyes, you admire it, discover it. You sample it in every possible way. You are in the moment. You're not thinking of what is going to happen next or what has happened in the past. You are just being you. You are letting your inner child play freely. You are carefree, comfortable in your own skin, no façade, honest as hell. (It's true! Look at every child around that age or younger, and they will tell you the honest truth without beating around the bush.) Do I need to continue? I think you get the picture, and you can imagine yourself back at that time.

And then we grow up and we lose the power of being real. This trait of unbiasedly being ourselves, of speaking our truth. We hide ourselves. We look at the world around us and conform ourselves to rules, beliefs, and values because we think it's the right thing for us. It'll keep us safe if we follow the mainstream. And don't get me wrong. A lot of those rules, beliefs, and values are indeed good for you; they shape a part of you. But when you arrive at a point where you feel lost, where you need to find the answer on who you really are deep down, where you notice you are hiding your true self just because you are afraid of what others might think or say when you don't follow those rules, then you are going down the rabbit hole. You are denying yourself the real you. You are not being authentic.

For me, 2010 and 2015 were huge pivotable moments regarding this matter (more about that later). These were years when my body and mind showed me (they screamed quite loudly, I must say) how I wasn't in tune with myself, how I didn't listen to my own inner voice anymore. I wasn't being authentic. I didn't trust my intuition, couldn't tap into it either, but I let others take over the reins. I trusted the values, beliefs, rules, and decisions of others more than my own. I wasn't true to myself.

In this chapter, I'd like to share what authenticity and intuition brought me as a human being, how it helped me health wise, how it helped me grow into being a better coach, how it formed my business, and how it helps my clients. Call it a strategy, a set of guiding principles or tools you can use as a life coach. I hope this strategy will help you and your clients tap into your authentic and intuitive power again.

Off-Road: What Happens When You Don't Listen to Your Own Voice

In 2010, after giving birth to my son, I had post-natal depression and a burnout. I don't remember much about that period, and when I look back on it today, I didn't learn from that life episode either. I just kept repeating the same patterns and ignored the signals my body gave me years after. I hadn't gained any insight as to why I was getting sick because five years later, in the fall of 2015, after I had changed jobs and had a new challenge, my energy was running out again. My batteries were completely drained. Burnout 2.0 was the verdict.

I had already experienced a burnout. How come I was having a second one now? Was this even possible? The reason: I hadn't listened to my own voice for years. I wasn't following my authentic path in life.

I did start on the right path when I studied assistant psychology. I loved everything around the human psyche, the research, the analysis, but courses you had to learn by heart like law were extremely hard for me. My statistics teacher told me I would have to work twice as hard to get there and that it would take twice as long to graduate. I was young, looked up to her, and thought she had all the answers, so I quit college. I changed direction and graduated a few years later as a kindergarten teacher. I always wanted to do something in the social branch, so this worked for me. But life happened, I moved in with my boyfriend, and we were getting married; therefore, I needed a job. I started to work in telecommunication where I bought into the beliefs I grew up with. Namely, "If you work hard in life, you'll achieve great things," "Keep on going," and "Never quit if life gets tough."

I didn't quit. My body quit on me before I could. First burnout in 2010 and burnout 2.0 in 2015. I wasn't being true to myself. I went for positions that didn't give me energy but gave me status, prestige, and validation. And, yes, working hard is a value that I maintain to this day, but now I follow this value on my own terms and guard it with my own boundaries. Back then, I thought (yes, "thought"—it all starts in our head) I would receive permission, validation of who I was by following the beliefs my parents gave me while I grew up. I had my own voice but didn't follow it out of fear of not being enough. What eventually led to a burnout was trying to gain that permission and feeling depressed because I didn't follow my own inner voice.

If I had learned to listen better to my inner voice, my intuition on my second job, I would have chosen much more quickly to quit the job that didn't match the person I was. Yup, already after a few weeks, my intuition told me that the job wasn't something for me. Still, I endured it, made the best of it, and eventually worked at that firm for almost 11 years because of a belief I grew up with.

The What: Be Intuitively Authentic

While looking up the meaning of "authenticity," this description resonated the most with me: being authentic = being true to yourself; you live life as the person you think yourself to be. You are open about your intentions and feelings while staying true to your values and beliefs.

You are you. You are here for a reason, and that's why you're special and unique in your own kind of way. It's all about not trying to fit yourself in the crowd. You are not here to impress others. And I know, it takes courage, vulnerability, faith, and self-awareness to put yourself out there, to be authentic. But it is so worth it.

> *The only real valuable thing is intuition.*
> —ALBERT EINSTEIN

What is intuition? And how do you know it's intuition?

Intuition—aka a hunch, instinct, perception, inner voice, or even your sixth sense—it's the ability you have to understand or know something without needing any proof, evidence, or use of reason.

For example: You are taking a shower and then all of a sudden, a friend's name pops up, you feel you need to reach out, but you don't know why. So you send out a text or even call your friend, and they say, "How did you know I was feeling off?" You didn't. You just had a hunch.

So what has intuition got to do with authenticity?

When you are being authentic, you are putting less stress on how to live your life; it leads you to where you should be according to what feels true and consistent with your beliefs and your identity. And this is where intuition pops up.

When you are more aware of yourself and you are listening to your inner voice, you are opening yourself up. Decisions, choices, answers are rising up from within. You don't know where it comes from, but your gut feeling guides you. Tapping into that power can be a great asset during your coaching sessions too.

The Why: Experience It

> *Be so authentically you that others*
> *feel safe to be themselves too.*
>
> —UNKNOWN

Having a strong "why" helps you with your goals; it gives you direction and motivation. So, if you are not yet convinced on why this will help you as a person or as a coach, these are results I experienced myself and with my clients when I was being authentic and listened to my intuition:

Energy saver: Since I don't need to put on a mask, I keep a lot of energy that I would lose otherwise by pretending to be someone I'm not.

State of flow: By being myself, being comfortable in my own skin during sessions, I'm not thinking of what's to come or what has passed. I'm just in the moment with my client. This also helps me to tap into my intuition much more easily. I'm not thinking of the next question to ask, nor do I follow a framework. In that moment, my mind is alert and focused on the person in front of me. The right questions, ideas, and exercises that my client needs just pop up in that moment.

Going deeper: I'm honest, open, and share my own obstacles, challenges, mistakes, and learning curves as examples throughout the sessions. I'm equal to the person that sits in front of me. I am not more or less than them. Through this, my clients feel they aren't alone on their path, which helps in building trust and confidence, which leads to greater self-motivation, a boost of energy that makes change happen.

Solid relationships: Being authentic also helps to build a strong and long relationship, sometimes even lasting ones. I have clients coming back years later to get more coaching, so they can jump onto that next level of growth for themselves. Some of them check in regularly with life updates even if they are no longer being coached.

Build your tribe: By showing the real you, you attract the right kind of people. People see who you are deep down, and if they like that, they're attracted to your energy. I have my ideal clients who come to me because they know who I am and what I stand for. My intuition will tell me if someone is not the right fit. This gives me the capacity to address this in a session and to redirect the person to a more aligned coach.

Increased happiness: By being the real me, I feel in sync with myself, I feel happy with who I am deep down and look positively at my life. This radiates onto my clients. They receive a space where they are welcome, feel at home, are not judged, and feel seen, a space where they can be vulnerable and be themselves.

Innate intelligence: When attuning more and more to your intuition, you are becoming aware of books, articles, conversations, people, and experiences that cross your path before a coaching session even takes place. For example, hours before a coaching session, I could've had a similar conversation or situation, even an article that popped up in my inbox that could guide the person in front of me. Questions related to an article I just read often pop up during a session and as a result, I am better able to give insight or stimulate growth for my client. Call it strange? For me, it's an innate intelligence I can tap from.

The How: Trust the Process

> *Don't trade who you are for who you think the world needs because the world needs you to be YOU.*
>
> —Jay Shetty

How to Practice Tapping into Your Own Intuition

Try these three scenarios for yourself and see what happens within yourself:

1. Prepare your next session thoroughly and follow the steps or frameworks you learned in coaching school.
2. Prepare the big lines of your session (e.g., reread your client's backstory, review the past session) and just go with this information into your session.
3. Don't prepare for your session. Go with the flow.

Try these three scenarios for yourself. With the same client or throughout different coaching sessions. Be aware of what pops up in your head (it can be questions, answers, directions, experiences), listen to your body (it can be a nudge in your stomach, a twitching nerve, a cold sensation going through your body), and focus your attention on your client (what they are saying and not saying, what their body language is telling you, what kind of energy you are feeling).

Don't look for answers, don't try to reason it with your mind; just be aware in the moment. Notice the difference in feeling with each session but also look for the difference in outcome for yourself and for your client.

For me, when I'm using scenario two or three, my client has more insights and the session flows fluently. My client is more motivated to make a change because they tapped into their authentic power; they made the decision by listening to their intuition in that moment.

While with scenario one, my client feels more guided and is leaning more on me instead of letting the solutions come from within. Most of the time, I even have an off feeling after such a kind of session, like it was blocked in a way.

What helps you to listen more easily to your intuition? Here are a few things I do that can be useful to you:

- Before each session, I take some time for myself to get in the flow. I go for a pitstop, open up my windows, and breathe. Sometimes I even put on a playlist to set myself in the right kind of mood. A calm state versus an agitated, stressed one will help you listen much better to that inner voice.
- Have enough sleep. If you are mentally off due to a lack of sleep, you will notice fewer things than if you are fully rested.
- Drink enough water. The brain is made of 70% water, so replenishing on time helps you to focus more clearly as well as being in the moment.

You don't need permission for being who you are. Just be you and the world will follow. Not the other way around.

ACTIVITY

See Tapping into Your Own Intuition within the chapter.

About the Author

Julie Stévigny is a coach and founder of the Happy Mind Guide. She specializes in guiding women who feel inadequate and overloaded to feel confident and energetic again.

Before starting as a coach, Julie gained her experience in various fields such as education, telecom, waste management, and transportation. Through these experiences, along with her own burnouts and mental challenges, she saw and experienced first hand that stress management is a challenge for many, as is taking good care of ourselves and listening to our authentic intuitive voice. Julie now guides people to create their own manual for a life with more energy, less stress, and a happy mind.

It's Julie's mission to guide others on their path to becoming the person they are destined to be, by helping them to reconnect with their true self while optimising their health. That's why she founded the Happy Mind House. A community where you're welcome, a house to resource and reconnect with your true inner self. Happy Mind House offers a variety of therapies, workshops, and trainings for body, mind, and soul.

Tapping into her own authentic power helped her change direction in life. She started her own company, founded a community, and wrote her first novel, all in a range of five years. So, what are you waiting for?

Email: julie@happymindguide.be
Website: www.happymindguide.be
Facebook: facebook.com/happymindguide.be, facebook.com/happymindhouse
Instagram: @happymindguide, @happymindhouse
LinkedIn: www.linkedin.com/in/julie-stévigny-aba423222

CHAPTER 25

The EM Dash

By Diana Usher
All About We, LLC
Lifestyle Management Coach
Oklahoma, USA

The only true wisdom is knowing that you know nothing.
—SOCRATES

Socrates' philosophy will lead to the path of least resistance in helping to find a person's True North. The more we know, the more we understand there is so much more to learn. How do we balance and expertly maintain all the sectors in our life?

As life coach experts, we take on the challenge of being a boss at being our own boss. And we do so while helping others master managing their own lives. If we present ourselves as experts of life management, the caveat is the implied pressure to flawlessly uphold this position, knowingly, both personally and professionally. This expectation can create feelings of inadequacy or trigger bouts of imposter syndrome. To strategically counter this destructive behavior is to simply present ourselves as transparently and vulnerably as possible. Building up personal branding and public relations involves connecting to others with our imperfect lives to demonstrate that all lives are a work in progress with both setbacks and successes.

The lives of life coaches are not perfect and actually shouldn't be. How can others relate to that high of an unobtainable level of existence? How will anyone resonate with a person having no issues? We are all human, we sometimes get upset, we make mistakes, we try new things, achieve goals, and at times we fail forward, trying new ways.

There is an anonymous quote, "If you learn to laugh at yourself, you'll never cease to be amused." Those who live by this notion can laugh at the paradox. We've all been there in that comical slapstick that we inadvertently get placed in. Where the more we try to control a mishap, the more mishaps occur. More often than not, it's more fun to find the humor in these circumstances. Joie de vivre! It's not only about waiting for the perfect day to find joy; it's also about finding joy during challenging storms.

It is such a freeing thought process to be unabashedly flawed. Mistakes happen, we aren't any more perfect than the people who seek our help. However, we are skilled, highly trained, and knowledgeable. We have studied, conversed with colleagues, gained experience, tried different approaches, methods, and modalities. We have a passion quest to keep learning about managing life. There is this visceral drive to relay this information in our unique ways because we desire for everyone to level up. We gain rewards by being a part of witnessing first-hand people putting into practice our coaching guidance to have their definition of success realized.

As entrepreneurs, we are on an ongoing quest to increase our knowledge, find new ideas, and build upon our offerings. Part of life is evolving, and with this growth, we will try and at times fail. We cannot set sail if we remain tied to the dock. Develop a plan, get some bearings, pull the anchor up, and cast off. Trying as a novice is an integral part of becoming an expert.

Transformation will happen. The one constant in life is that it is forever changing. How we evolve during these changes can be detrimental or instrumental towards the outcomes of our life's purpose when facing both shortcomings and successes. Every year will bring different challenges to face.

My grandma, Ruby, loved life; she would say that the golden years are in every year because each year provides golden memories. She taught me about LIL—LIL: Living is learning and learning is living. We cannot have one without the other. LIL—LIL is a growth mindset in understanding life is to be sought in the continuous pursuit of becoming our better self in both good times and bad. We are to become one another's teachers yet be mindful and alert in understanding that we are also one another's students. We will be learning what to do, and from some, learning what not to do. We absorb these encounters to either create ripples or break them.

It is up to us to decide how we will navigate these uncharted waters and convert these lessons into making our desired pursuits. And so, as we navigate throughout the course of our lives, we learn to ride these different waves. However, riding waves without relief is strenuous. Understand the power of the pause. Be still and float in the calm waters before setting course again. LIL—LIL is the art of inward cultivation by learning with a growth mindset, incorporating humility and gratitude.

Life Course 101 Session A and the Requisite Lab: Life Crash Course 101 Session B

Life Course 101 Session A is of our choosing. The world is ours to explore in delight to learn and grow. We can seek out new ventures with no time demarcations. Life can be exhilarating! It is our time to go out in the world with the heart of a child at play. It can be exciting and fun with anxious anticipation of discovering new things, tantalizing our senses and often presented with serendipitous surprises.

These are times when perhaps we are experiencing new jobs, new logistics, new homes, a new partner, having a baby, new fur baby, new crafts, new excursions, graduating, pursuing degrees or certificates, or life experiences that build our career skillset. We try new experiences to titillate our sensory processing. We find passions, partners, friends, new hobbies, practiced disciplines, learning exercise, sport, dieting, reading new books, or attending new seminars, etc.

With each moment, cherishing amazing circumstances when something comes that has everything fall perfectly into place. We are exuberant as our heart dances with joy and gratitude. It encompasses chartering new beginnings and seeing the best in what life has to offer.

The EM Dash

Embrace these rays of sunshine and blue skies. It's easy to flow when life is carefree. We smile, laugh, and engage with a positive mindset.

However, staying on top of the crest of this wave can be deceptively too easy and somewhat addicting. Some will dare to fly off too high toward the sun, melting their wings in the rush to recapture or increase the highs, in perpetual pursuit of dopamine energy and adrenaline rushes. While others relive the dazzling high via repetitive memory recall until it loses its luster to then becomes dulled. Some will fall into discontentment, leading to boredom, and for some, depression.

Additionally, and unfortunately inevitably, life also brings unexpected forces that redirect us against our will.

Crash Course 101 Session B, conversely, is exhausting and exacting. These are the breaker waves. It is when life happens upon us. Sometimes with such horrific force, it traps us in the undertow, with complete wipeouts.

It knocks us so hard; it shakes the very being of who we are. It sucks the life out of us and makes us reevaluate our values. The plunge plummets us to the depths of despair, tormenting our psyche with doubts of desire to continue on.

It pulls us into fetal position to draw our knees up into our chest, breaks us down, and takes our breath. The heart pain is so sharp it would seem strong enough to kill us if but from one more inhale.

These tidal waves come in different forms, from unexpected deaths of loved ones, life-threatening diseases and disabilities, abrupt divorces, financial ruin, betrayal... It is an unwanted, uninvited cataclysmic life-altering event.

For myself, I have had plenty rip tides knock me down. One that was shockingly harsh and swift was the loss of my loving boyfriend, Gary, and six good crew mates.

I found solace by consoling family and friends. What I did not realize was that as I was trying to lift others and create an appearance of holding my own, I was, all the while, slowly sinking into a depressive state of mind. I was living life going through the motions of functionality.

The epiphany to snap out of it came from when I was sitting in the living room in a vegetative state, drawing further into my reclusive inner world. I remember thinking I had listlessly answered something I thought would suffice for my four-year-old grandson's question—evidently not.

With a stark disruption in thought, a rambunctious old soul, my little Cameron, decisively and clumsily climbed up onto my lap. He willfully cupped his two little hands to press my cheeks in, forcefully pushed his forehead on to mine, gave me a good hard eye-to-eye stare down, and with profound wisdom declared, "I'm here, Nana!" This little twister made his own cyclonic shift. And with the biggest bear hugs succeeded by tickles and giggles, I gladly exclaimed, "Yes, you are!" This moment was the catalyst to transport me into the now, to remind me to live life with gratitude for all my loved ones here and present in my life.

Many of us go through the ebb and flow, fluctuating our focus on the highs and lows. We tend to draw energy from them and aim our future plans based on the learned emotions with these past experiences. Depending upon the fear or the elation, it sets the framework of our mind to make headway.

This mindset of moving without purpose, bobbing up and down may eventually lead to feeling lost at sea with no thoughts of which direction to take, like a spinning compass. The mind, body, and spirit become quite exhausted staying in the crests and troughs. We can get motion sickness in either attempting to steer straight into these choppy waters or get stubbornly dependent on remaining in either high or low tides. There comes a point where many need an anchor to navigate through these extremes. This strength can come from family and friends, or often it may be a time to seek outside connections from professionals. Most times a therapist would come into play when a victim is drowning. They are in need of intensive support for complex or chronic trauma with long-term treatment. Life coaches are typically sought after for acute trauma when people are treading. They need a ring buoy tossed to get back onboard with some helpful measures for positioning and setting coordinates to set sail again.

People have been led astray looking at the wrong maps, either by asking and/or listening to others that may not know the right course to take, by looking backwards to the past, or haphazardly chasing what's in front of them.

With life coaching, the ethereal moment is when we can help others to realize at times it is when we are at our weakest moments, we find our deepest strengths. And the way to finding our True North is to stop moving.

This is represented by the em dash in LIL—LIL. Although small, this punctuation mark is the ever so important connector of both Session A and B. It is the purposeful breaking of the normal thought process in order to maintain a healthy lifestyle. This significant pause allows us to recenter and gain back our equilibrium.

A life coach can utilize one or several methodologies to help a client to bring back the focus to chart a new course by directing them to look within. It is understanding that this is a vital component to execute—regularly—for this inward focus is the safe haven to replenish and fortify. In these calm waters, the mind and body slow down. This is when needs assessment can be discovered. By listening to our breath and heartbeat, and quieting the ego, our higher self can re-energize to build power and strength in self-efficacy. This stillness can be guided, for example, in religious faith, spiritual beliefs, meditation, nature grounding, therapy, and coaching.

Highs and lows are an integral part of life, yet so too is the precious time to pause in between. There is as much value, if not more, by maintaining and appreciating life at a level status. The ability of going within is a place of equanimity and is our safe harbor. This is where our inner student transitions to teacher in becoming our better self.

In one of his bestselling books, *The Power of Now*, renowned philosophist and author, Eckhart Tolle, teaches us to live in the present. Accept the now. When we begin to live in a state of present mindset, we do not react either positively or negatively; we experience it, thus becoming the captain of our ship. Our maneuvers become intentional. We become empowered by the acknowledgement of the present moment for what it is. Accepting the moment intrinsically without confusion from the ego. We can learn from our past and yet still detach emotionally from it so that we can move forward effectively.

When we resist or avoid the present, we become a water-gate, blocked, potentially leading to bursting.

Bruce Lee, martial artist, actor, and philosopher expressed eloquently a tactic that many life coaches use. It is about becoming transformative. He explains in an interview, "Empty your mind, be formless, shapeless like water. You put water into a cup, it becomes the cup. You put it into a bottle, it becomes the bottle. You put it in a teapot, it becomes the teapot. Now water can flow or it can crash. Be water, my friend."

As life coaches, we have the gamut of resources to delve into, refining our unique techniques and styles by expanding our comprehension in EQ, PQ, AQ, SQ, and more.

Diverse studies are abundant with well renowned certifications for life coaches, business management consultants, company motivators, instructional performance educators. We can choose to learn about growth models, develop extensive questionnaires, articulate content with values, boundaries, and non-negotiables. Life coaching can include a spiritual journey of the coachee connecting with the inner child, figuratively and literally. Perhaps incorporating Viktor Frankl's logotherapy practices, aligning it with the Greek concepts of symbolic elements: soma (body/earth), psyche (mind/water: air), and noos (spirit/fire). A life coach could choose to traverse to focus on shamanic rituals, crystals, and animal spirits.

Life coaches have a wide spectrum of research to take a deep dive in establishing the direction, niche, and style by finding clarity through their own stillness, purposeful listening, and intent. We are enlightened that growth has no boundaries. The more we learn in honing our skillset, the more we understand what course we will take, the more we are exposed to finding there is so much more to learn. Celebrate the quest of continuous self-improvement as this becomes invaluable for ourselves and improves the value of what we have to offer.

As life coaches, we get to be honored by creating relationships that connect and resonate with our unique, personal style. By others choosing and placing us at the helm with their transparency and vulnerability, we become vessels of servant leadership. Success thrives from inner cultivation. This purpose of intentional kindness inwardly generates the inertia to create outward movement, serenely to avoid creating wakes. However our inspired style flows from, it always begins from within. Self-awareness leads to self-empowerment, which leads to successful relationships and endeavors. Rest assured, kind reciprocity returns tenfold.

We embark on cultivating self-love—"All About Me"—then launch out to love exponentially—"All About We."

As life coaches, we are mapping out our own expeditions to become captains of our own ships. And with time and experience, we transform from being new journeymen getting our sea legs to seasoned admirals in assisting other captains. Coaching styles are as big as the ocean because each coach is unique, and each style will resonate to others because of our uniqueness. What we have in common is the desire to guide everyone to become their best. We stay thirsty for the quest of continuous improvement. We understand and embody the principle meaning of the phrase, "Together we rise."

Fair winds and following seas: bon voyage!

ACTIVITY

Name:		*Symbol:*
Values	**Boundaries**	**Non-Negotiables**
Choose five values important enough to set standards to focus on and live by.	Set physical, mental, and emotional parameters to protect and keep these values intact.	Create actions to ensure values are not at risk of being impeded.
I.		
II.		
III.		
IV.		
V.		

There are many values to live by. However, choosing five to focus on will enable a more concentrated focus.

All About We, LLC

The EM Dash

Here is a list of core values *(not in its entirety)*.
Naturally, we all have these attributes to some degree.
What five values resonate as most important for internal well-being?

ACCEPTANCE	FAIRNESS	LEADERSHIP	SELF-LOVE
ACCOMPLISHMENT	FAITH	LEARNING	SELF-RESPECT
ACCOUNTABILITY	FAMILY	LOGIC	SELFLESS
ADAPTABILITY	FITNESS	LOVE	SERVICE
AMBITION	FOCUS	LOYALTY	SOLITUDE
AWARENESS	FRIENDSHIP		SPIRITUALITY
		MASTERY	STRENGTH
BALANCE	GENEROSITY	MODERATION	SUSTAINABILITY
BEAUTY	GOODNESS	MOTIVATION	SUCCESS
BELONGING	GRACE		
BRAVERY	GRATITUDE	OPENNESS	TEAMWORK
	GROWTH-MINDSET	OPTIMISM	TEMPERANCE
CALMNESS		ORGANIZATION	THANKFUL
CAPABLE	HEALTH	ORIGINALITY	TOLERANCE
CAREFUL	HONESTY		TRADITIONAL
COMPASSION	HONOR	PASSION	TRANQUILITY
CREATIVITY	HUMILITY	PLAYFULNESS	TRANSPARENCY
	HUMOR	POSITIVITY	TRUSTWORTHY
DEPENDABILITY		POWER	
DETERMINATION	INSPIRING	PURPOSE	UNDERSTANDING
DIGNITY	INTEGRITY		UNIQUENESS
DISCIPLINE	INTELLIGENCE	QUALITY	UNITY
DIVERSITY	INTUITIVE		
		RECOGNITION	VISION
ENERGY	JOY	RESPECT	VITALITY
QUALITY	JUSTICE	RESPONSIBILITY	
ETHICAL		RESULTS-	WEALTH
EXPERIENCE	KINDNESS	ORIENTED	WELCOMING
EXECUTION	KNOWLEDGE		WISDOM

All About We, LLC

About the Author

As an altruist, Diana Usher enjoys projects that provide impactful differences in assisting others. She listens and learns about an individual's thought process, their experiences, talents, and back story — assessing needs factors to develop strategies for successful living that is congruent with their authentic well-being.

Diana's professional quest is fulfilled by being in alignment with working as a Family Services Specialist II for OKDHS, a consultant for World Financial Group, and as a Transformation Academy, Life Purpose certified, lifestyle management coach for her precious business gem, All About We, LLC.

Diana's personal and spiritual passions involve nature, writing, painting, sculpting, dancing, reading, researching, continuous education "Go SOSU Savage Storm!", and takes pleasure in creating lovely human connections.

It would be remiss with introductions without mentioning a huge part of who she is in being a grateful mom to Amanda and Sarah, nana to Ian, Nickolas, and Cameron, little sis to Arabel, heart-adopted mom to Brandon and Alexa, auntie, niece, cousin, and akin to her high-vibe tribe, Renata, Sandi, Juliana, Sheila, Lance and many more lovely kindreds.

She finds it priceless to see eyes light up when the inner spirit fully embraces life and all it has to offer. "To live abundantly, the first dance must be solo, then we can leap into the rhythm of our outer world to blend in harmony with others".

Email: diana@allaboutwe.live
LinkedIn: https://www.linkedin.com/in/diana-usher/

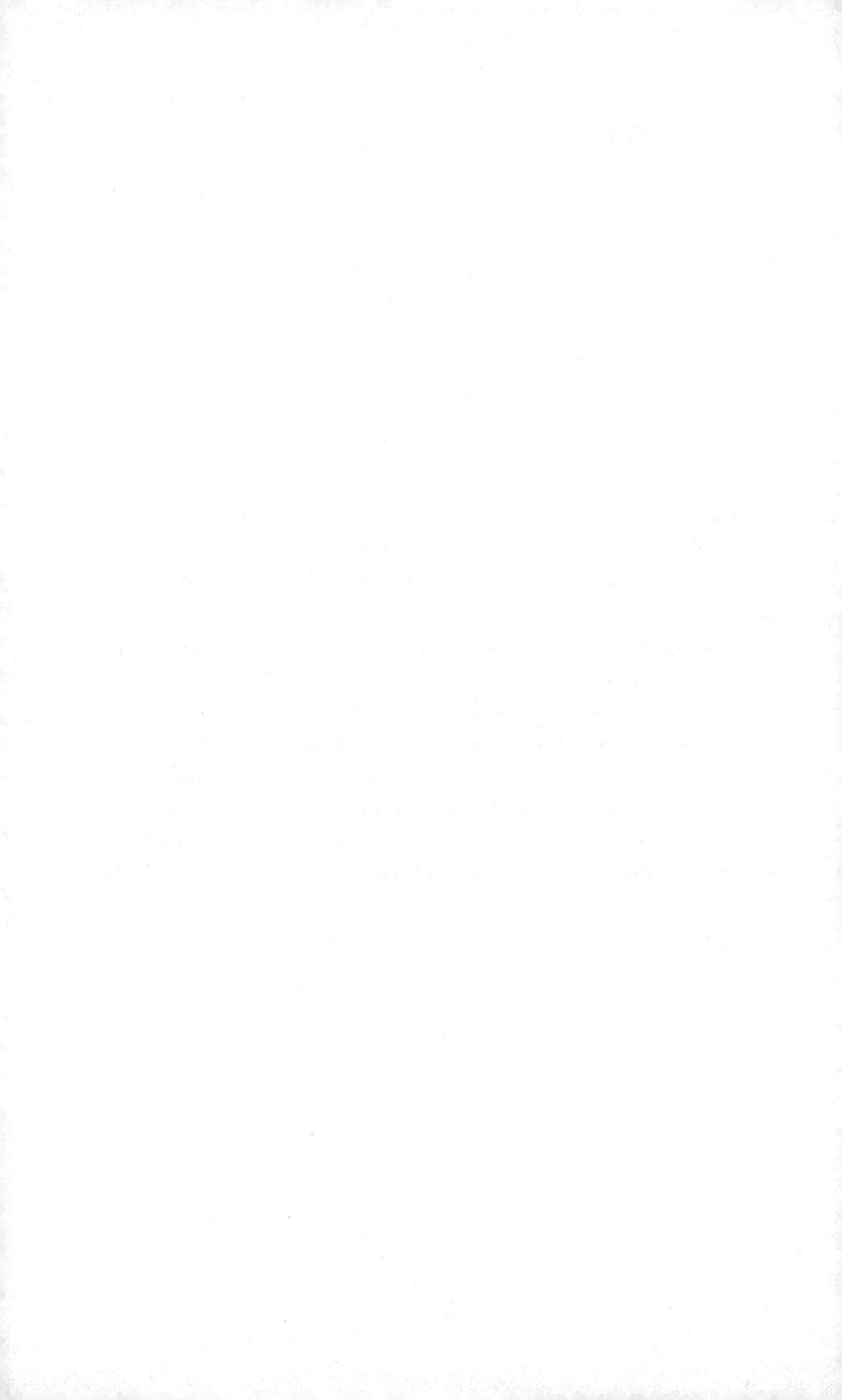

DID YOU ENJOY THIS BOOK?

If you enjoyed reading this book, you can help by suggesting it to someone else you think might like it, and **please leave a positive review** wherever you purchased it. This does a lot in helping others find the book. We thank you in advance for taking a few moments to do this.

THANK YOU

You might also like other Thin Leaf Press titles:

The Life Coach's Tool Kit, Vol 1
The Successful Mind: Tools to Living a Purposeful, Productive, and Happy Life
The Successful Body: Using Fitness, Nutrition, and Mindset to Live Better
The Successful Spirit: Top Performers Share Secrets to a Winning Mindset
Winning Mindset: Elite Strategies for Peak Performance
Winner's Mindset: Peak Performance Strategies for Success
Peak Performance: Mindset Tools for Sales
Peak Performance: Mindset Tools for Leaders
Peak Performance: Mindset Tools for Business
Peak Performance: Mindset Tools for Entrepreneurs
Peak Performance: Mindset Tools for Athletes
Ordinary to Extraordinary
Explore.

Made in United States
Orlando, FL
30 April 2024